PM&R Recap

PM&R Recap
Companion Text

Alexander D'Angelo, M.D.

Alexander D'Angelo, M.D.

ISBN: 9781672358583

Table of Contents

Chapter 1: Introduction to PM&R

PM&R Recap

- This educational series is intended to serve as a high-yield PM&R board review course
- It's also intended to prepare medical students, residents, and fellows for various PM&R rotations
- Attending physicians may find this course useful to brush up on their knowledge or prepare for recertification
  - To recap, if you will
- The goal here is high-yield PM&R information without any extra fluff
- Only what you need to know, and nothing else, to do well on exams, on rotations, and in practice

PM&R Core Concepts

- The goal of PM&R physicians (physiatrists) is to maintain or improve the **function** of patients with disabilities, notably with regard to their activities of daily living (ADLs)
- **Impairment:** loss of a structure or function
  - Foot drop (can't raise foot)
- **Disability:** essentially the inability to perform ADLs
  - Inability to ambulate
- **Participation/Handicap:** participation in society
  - Cannot climb the stairs to reach office at work
- *Function* is the organ system of PM&R physicians

PM&R Scope of Practice

- PM&R physicians enjoy a wide range of clinical practices and settings
- Inpatient, outpatient, procedural-based, academic, private practice, and every combination thereof
- Subspecialties and fellowships are numerous
  - Traumatic brain injury (TBI)
  - Neurorehab (e.g. stroke)
  - Spinal cord injury (SCI)
  - Sports medicine
  - Pain medicine
  - Sports and spine
  - Cancer rehab
  - Regenerative medicine

- ○ EMG
- ○ Pediatric rehab

PM&R Scope of Practice

- PM&R physicians are experts of the neuromusculoskeletal system
- In residency you learn how to accurately diagnose and treat various disorders of the neuro-MSK system
- **Diagnosis** via physical exam, imaging (xray, CT, MRI, ultrasound) electrodiagnostic studies (EMG/NCS), blood and urine studies
- **Treatment** via physical, occupational, and speech therapy, targeted exercise, modalities, medications, injections, and various other interventions
- Everything is geared toward improving the patient's function

PM&R Treatments

- **Therapeutic exercise**
  - ○ The exercise prescription from a physiatrist should be detailed with specific instructions on what needs to be done
  - ○ Type of exercise, frequency (how often), intensity (how hard), duration, # sets, # repetitions (reps), open chain vs. closed chain, concentric vs. eccentric focus, isometric vs. isotonic vs. isokinetic, and...any precautions (e.g. sternal precautions due to sternal fracture)
  - ○ Important to specify, because often patients will tell you they "tried PT, but it didn't work", and they just weren't doing the right type of exercises for a long enough time

Types of Exercises

- **Isometric:** no movement occurs
  - ○ Planks, wall sits, pushing against a wall, flexing your muscles in the mirror
- **Isotonic:** tone pulling on the muscle is the same
  - ○ Biceps curls
- **Isokinetic:** the movement and rhythm of the exercise is constant
  - ○ Cardio machines: elliptical, bike, rowing

Types of Muscle Fibers

- **Type I Muscle Fibers**
  - ○ "One slow, red ox"
    - ■ Type I, slow twitch, "red" muscle, +ox-phos (aerobic)
  - ○ EMG generally just picks up Type I fibers

- **Type II Muscle Fibers**
  - Type II, fast twitch, "white" muscle, anaerobic
    - The opposite of Type I fibers
    - Only picked up and analyzed on EMG with maximal contraction
    - Type IIa = mixed glycolytic and aerobic
    - Type IIb = pure glycolytic (anaerobic)
      - E.g. sprinting, powerlifting

Aerobic Exercise

- **Aerobic exercise** is good for the heart and lungs
  - This is not because it works the heart and lungs
  - Rather, it is because it conditions the peripheral musculature to do a better job of oxygen uptake
  - When the peripheral muscles soak up more of the oxygen that's being delivered from the blood, the heart doesn't need to pump as much blood their direction
  - Thus, the heart slows down and you breathe more slowly, because the muscles take up plenty of oxygen from what "little" blood gets sent their way
  - Running, treadmill, elliptical, rowing, swimming, stair-climbing, etc. are all good aerobic exercises

- Water aerobics are beneficial for pain, especially OA-related pain
  - This is not a weight-bearing exercise, however, so not great for osteoporosis
- The American College of Sports Medicine (ACSM) recommends patients achieve 150 minutes of moderate aerobic exercise per week

Muscle Contraction

- **Concentric contraction** = the muscle shortens as it contracts against a load
  - E.g curling the dumbbell up while doing a biceps curl
- **Eccentric contraction** = the muscle lengthens as it fights to contract against this
  - E.g. slowly lowering the dumbbell back down to your waist level
- Eccentric contraction tends to be the most useful in therapy programs for muscle-building and tendon health
- Fast, eccentric contractions put the most stress on the tendon
  - Highest risk for tendon rupture

Progressive Resistance Exercises

- PREs invoke the idea that in order for a motor unit and the muscle to adapt and grow stronger with better control and more precise firing patterns, the athlete/patient needs to progressively add weight to the exercise to make it harder

- The muscle must "grow or die"
- The muscle must be challenged if you want it to adapt
- PREs are sometimes called "DeLorme's exercises"

Biofeedback in Exercise

- Biofeedback is the principle of utilizing some type of sensory input to augment exercise
  - Useful in patients with motor and sensory impairments (stroke, TBI, SCI, etc.)
- Feedback can be touch, visual, audio, EMG biofeedback, breathing-related, etc.

Muscle Physiology

- Muscle cells are called myocytes
- Each myocyte has lots of sarcomeres within it
- Sarcomeres are the structures in muscle cells that contract
- When lots and lots of sarcomeres contract at the same time, the muscle shortens
- Actin and myosin are long structures that overlap like interlocking fingers
- When a muscle is contracting, myosin binds to actin and pulls the two actin structures towards each other, like interlocking fingers moving towards each other
- The sarcomere has H zone, Z line, I band, A band

Modalities in Therapy

- Modalities are interventions that augment a therapy program using some kind of energy directed toward the patient's body
- This can be heat, ice, ultrasound, diathermy, soundwaves, pressure, electricity/stimulation, light

Heat

- Heat therapy can be transmitted via direct skin contact (conduction), via a flowing fluid (convection), or via radiation (conversion)
- Conduction: heat pads
- Convection: whirlpool
- Conversion: heat lamp
- Heat is useful to loosen structures up for improved ROM and for comfort
- Do not use heat over electrical implants (pacemaker), cancer, infection, or over insensate areas, skin damage, DVT

Cold

- Cold works by the same heat transfer principles of conduction and convection

- Conduction: cold packs

- Convection: cold whirlpool

- Cold is useful for pain (decreases metabolism and blood flow on that area)

- Do not use cold over areas of skin breakdown, insensate skin, PVD

Ultrasound and Diathermy

- **Ultrasound** = ultrasonic frequency sound waves above the range of our hearing bombard the skin structures underneath it with constant sound waves that produce vibrations that heat up these deeper tissues
  - ~1 MHz
  - Great for heating tendons (tendonitis), pain, ligaments, up to 8 cm deep
  - Do not use near electrical implants or cancer

- **Short wave diathermy** = radio waves bombard the tissues to heat them up
  - ~27 MHz
  - Great for more superficial structures up to 5 cm deep
  - Do not use over metal, over a pregnancy, etc.

- **Microwave diathermy** = microwaves that heat very superficial structures
  - ~1000 MHz
  - Great for superficial structures 1-3 cm deep such as hematomas
  - Do not use over metal, over a pregnancy, cancer, etc.

Phonophoresis

- Uses sound waves to blast medication through the skin and deeper tissues in order to reach a target structure

- Usually inject lidocaine and corticosteroids into superficial structures such as the achilles tendon

Pressure Modality

- AKA massage, traction, manual techniques

- Feels good, improves psychological state

- Massage techniques

- Manual therapy techniques
  - Muscle energy: isometric contractions followed by stretching
  - Myofascial release: stretch the heck out of a muscle so that the muscle and fascia are no longer tight

- Traction
  - Traction can be useful to pull the vertebrae apart to relieve pressure on the nerve roots
    - Do not perform if patient has spinal infection or cancer, ligamentous instability, VBI

Electricity / Stimulation

- Iontophoresis, transcutaneous nerve stimulation (TENS), and neuromuscular electrical stimulation (NMES) are all helpful uses of electricity

Electricity / Stimulation

- **Iontophoresis** = use electricity to drive medicated ions through the skin and towards a target structure
  - E.g. achilles tendon

Electricity / Stimulation

- **TENS (transcutaneous nerve stimulation)**
  - Electrodes are placed onto the patient's skin, usually over the area of pain
  - The electrodes supply electricity directly into the skin
  - The Gate Control Theory kicks in and decreases the patient's pain

- **The Gate Control Theory of Pain**
  - Light touch and pressure neurons (large Ia/ A Beta sensory neurons) synapse onto the same layer in the substantia gelatinosa as pain fibers do (C fibers)
  - If lots and lots of light touch/pressure sensations are occurring on the skin, they can actually inhibit any pain signals coming in at that level from the pain fibers (C fibers)
    - This is why when you fall and have a knee scrape, it feels better when you rub it

Electricity / Stimulation

- **NMES (neuromuscular electrical stimulation)**
  - Stimulate motor nerves to contract muscles
  - This helps with biofeedback in patients learning to use these muscles again and restore proper motor patterns
  - Either a therapist can trigger the contraction or a more complicated system can be installed to do this
  - Good for muscle-building, motor training, circulation, fitness

Light Therapy

- Ultraviolet radiation can be used mostly for skin conditions

- ○ Psoriasis uses UV light to treat plaques
- ○ Can help wound healing and kill bacteria

Wheelchairs and Assistive Devices
- Durable medical equipment (DME) is bread and butter PM&R
- Wheelchairs are used by many different patient populations
  - ○ Can be manual or power
- Assistive devices are also used by many different patient populations
  - ○ Canes, walkers, crutches, etc.
- Let's talk about both of these categories

Wheelchairs

Wheelchair Components
- Wheels/Tires
- Caster wheels
- Handrim (pushrim)
- Axle
- Handles on back for pushing
- Back rest
- Arm rests
- Seat
- Cushion
- Hand brakes
- Foot plate
- Anti-tippers

Wheels and Tires
- **Spoke wheels** = lighter, but require more maintenance
- **Mag wheels** = heavier, more durable (more popular)
- **Pneumatic tires** = rubber with an inner air-filled tube
  - ○ Smooth, cushioned ride, better for carpets
  - ○ Can be popped and go flat
  - ○ Need to be refilled with air

- **Solid rubber tires** = solid rubber
  - Less smooth of a ride because you feel every bump
  - Will not go flat
  - Little if any maintenance

- **Caster wheels** = tiny wheels at the front of the wheelchair that allow for steering
  - Smaller casters = easier to maneuver and turn WC, but it will get caught on every pebble

Wheel Position and Camber Angle

- If rear wheels are placed more anteriorly
  - Easier to maneuver chair, smaller turning radius, easier to do wheelies and go up curbs
  - Less stable (which is the reason you can do wheelies in the first place)

- If rear wheels are placed more posteriorly
  - Harder to maneuver, accelerate, and ascend inclines
  - More stable

- Camber angle
  - The amount of inward lean that the wheels have
  - Huge camber angle means the tops of the wheels point inward toward your body
  - This allows for really tight turns (you will want this if playing competitive WC basketball!)
  - The disadvantage is that your chair is now a lot wider (the bottoms of the wheels stick out wider)

Wheelchair Handrim / Pushrim

- The handrim is the metal wheel just next to the tire that your hand is supposed to grip to allow you to propel the chair and roll the wheels

- If hemiplegic, you can install a handrim system that allows you to control both wheels using one arm

Wheelchair Axle

- The axle is the position on the wheelchair where your wheels will sit

- Essentially the center of the wheel being affixed to the chair

- The axle position can be adjusted, as discussed, to move the wheels posteriorly or anteriorly

Wheelchair Armrests

- Armrests are usually tubular, removable, desk-length
- Tubular is better for transfers than standard armrests
- Removable is better for transfers and storage
- Desk-length allows you to get closer to the sink, table, desk, etc.

Wheelchair Seat

- The seat can be either solid or vinyl sling
  - Solid = firm, good for putting a cushion on top of
  - Vinyl sling = cheap, good for transport wheelchair and folding/storage

Wheelchair Seat Cushions

- Seat cushions are important to provide comfort and prevent skin breakdown
- **Air villous** cushions are most popular
  - Require lots of maintenance, but are light and provide excellent pressure relief
- There are other types of cushions, such as foam, that are less popular, as they all do not provide as good of pressure relief as air villous does

Wheelchair Handbrakes

- Levers near the armrests that allow you to either push or pull on them in order to lock the wheels
- Pull-to-lock is more common, so that you don't accidentally unlock your wheels when trying to perform a transfer

Wheelchair Footplates

- Foot plates allow for the feet to rest
- They can be fixed in place or swing-away
- Swing-away is common due to allowing for easier transfers

Anti-Tippers

- Wheels in the far back of the wheelchair that, should the wheelchair be tipped backwards, will touch the ground and prevent the wheelchair from further tipping back and completely crashing
- Essentially they will catch you if you fall backward

Power Wheelchairs

- Similar components, only they are driven not by manual propulsion, but by power, usually via a joystick on the armrest
- You can also drive via head controls or sip and puff (breathing controls)

Measurements

- **Seat height** = distance from heel to posterior thigh when knee is bent 90°, plus a few inches to clear the floor, minus any extra padding (e.g. seat)

- **Seat width** = distance between the hips (+1 inch if using PWC)

- **Seat depth** = distance from pop fossa straight backward to the buttocks, minus 1/2 inch so that your pop fossae actually clear the seat and don't get compressed

- **Backrest height** = just below the bottom corner of the scapula (to the top/spine of the scapula if PWC)

- If things are too narrow or short, you risk putting too much pressure on the affected areas of skin

- If things are too wide or long, you risk compressing things (pop fossae) or simply not providing enough postural support (e.g. chair too wide)

Special Features of Wheelchairs

- Recline

- Tilt-in-Space

- Power Assist

Recline and Tilt-in-Space

- Recline = backrest reclines backward and allows you to lie flat
    - Good for opening up space to allow access for clean intermittent cath
    - Bad because it can increase shear forces on the posterior

- Tilt-in-Space = the entire chair keeps you in whatever seated position you are in while the whole thing tilts backward as one unit
    - Good for pressure relief and redistribution to prevent pressure injuries
    - Does not increase shear forces
    - More expensive

Power Assist for Manual Wheelchairs

- A power-generating device can be attached to the back of the chair and connect to the wheels

- With each manual stroke of the wheelchair during propulsion, the device sends power into the wheels that assists in rolling the wheels and accelerating the chair

- Enables you either go fast or go uphill with ease

Assistive Devices

- Canes, walkers, crutches

- All of these are used in order to widen a person's base of support so that they don't fall

Canes

- Canes are essentially poles used to widen a person's base of support
- They can also be used to unload painful limbs
  - Painful, arthritic hip or knee
- Canes can be straight or pronged
  - Straight cane is essentially a metal stick
  - Pronged canes can have 3 points of contact with the ground or 4 (quad cane)
  - Quad canes for example provide great support, but take up more space, are less maneuverable, and less fashionable
- Canes can be adjustable with different handle grip styles
- Cane height should be at the level of the greater trochanter, or the level of the hand when the elbow is flexed 20-30°

Walkers

- Walkers are essentially very broad canes
- They provide a much wider base of support and allow you to use your upper body to support yourself more so than canes
- They can be standard (pick up and put down), or wheeled (rolls along with you)
- Less fashionable, more "elderly"
- Good for leg weakness, pain, and instability (ALS, PD, stroke, cerebellar disease)

Crutches

- **Standard axillary crutches**
  - Grip for hands is midway down the crutch shaft
  - Do not apply pressure into your axillae; you're supposed to tense your triceps and keep your arms straight as you bear weight through your triceps, not your armpits
- **Lofstrand crutches (forearm crutches)**
  - Allow the forearms to bear the weight while it frees up your hands for ADLs, turning door handles, etc.
  - Less fashionable/socially acceptable

Congrats on finishing Chapter 1! You are well on your way to becoming the best physiatrist you can be.

Chapter 2: Stroke and Movement Disorders

Definition and Epidemiology of Stroke

- Interruption of blood supply to an area of the brain, causing signs and symptoms of intracranial neurologic compromise
  - Focal neurologic deficit, weakness, numbness, cranial nerve dysfunction, bowel/bladder dysfunction, etc.
  - If this occurs and signs/symptoms last for **under 24 hours, it is a TIA**
- ~85% are ischemic; ~15% are hemorrhagic
- Age is the most important risk factor
- HTN is the most important modifiable risk factor
- Old, African-American male is at highest nonmodifiable risk
- HTN, smoking, DM2, HLD, CAD/CHF, Afib, carotid stenosis are major risk factors
  - Systemic vascular disease is the common theme among these

Types of Stroke - Ischemic

- ~85% ischemic; ~15% hemorrhagic
- **Ischemic:** cutting off blood flow due to...
  - **Embolism:** usually heart throws a clot up to the brain (e.g. MCA)
    - Sudden-onset deficits
  - **Thrombosis:** systemic vascular disease from previous risk factors discussed produces a clot which grows and occludes the vessel lumen
    - Gradual-onset deficits
    - Most common ischemic stroke type
  - **Lacunar:** interruption of blood supply in the small lacunar vessels of the brain (**putamen,** thalamus, internal capsule)
    - Variable onset; related to **hypertension**

Types of Stroke - Hemorrhagic

- **Hemorrhagic:** a blood vessel bursts, leading to interruption of blood supply
- **Subarachnoid hemorrhage (SAH):** berry aneurysm bursts at the Circle of Willis (AComm)
  - Sudden-onset during exertion, "worst headache of my life"
  - **AComm** or PComm are most common sites
    - PComm aneurysm may cause CN 3 compression → blown pupil → ptosis, down and out
  - Patient in 40s-50s
  - Hunt and Hess Scale of 1-5
    - 1 = roughly asymptomatic

- 2 = headache, neck stiffness
- 3 = headache, neck stiffness, confused
- 4 = completely unintelligible as if they are very drunk, hemiparesis
- 5 = coma
  - These patients have increased acute mortality, but generally more favorable functional prognosis if they survive the acute period

Types of Stroke - Hemorrhagic

- **Intracerebral hemorrhage (ICH):** hypertension causes a vessel to burst
  - Sudden-onset while at rest; nausea, vomiting, seizures
  - **Putamen** is most common site
    - Contralateral hemiplegia

Acute Stroke Management

- Acute survey of the patient (airway, breathing, circulation) as these can become compromised in acute strokes
  - Secure airway (intubate if needed), make NPO, make bp not too high or too low
- Patient is now stable → stat head CT without contrast
  - Blood shows up bright white on head CT
  - Rules hemorrhage (ICH/SAH) in or out
- ASA 325 mg
- BP control with IV labetalol
  - Ischemic: keep SBP < 220
  - Hemorrhagic: keep SBP < 180
  - Permissive HTN with gradual return to normotension goals over next few weeks
- If seizure, give IV lorazepam → phenytoin/fosphenytoin

Acute Stroke Management

- **Keep ICP < 20 mmHg**
- Remember, **we want CPP to be > 60 mmHg** (most important point)
  - **CPP = MAP - ICP**
- Use forced hyperventilation, IV mannitol, elevate HOB, hypothermia, or perform neurosurgical Burr hole decompression (as last resort, or if there are signs of imminent decompensation)
- If ischemic, **consider tPA** if presenting within 3 hours of stroke onset, adult (not elderly), negative head CT for blood, SBP < 185, INR < 1.7, platelets > 100k, and stroke territory involves < 1/3 of the MCA territory

- If ischemic, consider thrombectomy

Acute Stroke Management

- If SAH/ICH
  - Commonly due to berry aneurysm rupture or AVM rupture
  - Major goal is to reduce any sort of strain on the patient that might increase bp
  - Keep SBP < 180
  - Keep stool soft (docusate, polyethylene glycol)
  - Keep ICP < 20
  - Give nimodipine x21 days to prevent secondary intracranial vasospasm due to blood irritating the vessels
  - Perform clipping/coiling of the aneurysm or removing the AVM

Imaging Studies

- Initial **head CT** without contrast
  - Blood is **bright white** on noncontrast head CT
  - Infarction is dark area (usually takes 1-2 days to show up)
- **MRI/MRA** with contrast/conventional angiography
  - The contrast allows us to view the neck and intracranial vasculature to look for AVMs/aneurysms/stenosis/occlusion
  - Blood is dark on T2 MRI
  - Infarction is **bright white** on T2 MRI (T2 = H20 = edema)
- Cardiac **echocardiogram** (TTE/TEE)
  - Look for cardiac embolus source / wall motion abnormalities/ PFO
- **Lumbar puncture**
  - Xanthochromia (blood breakdown products) can be detected, indicating SAH
  - Helpful when head CT is not informative but you still suspect SAH
- **Carotid artery US**
  - Can be helpful to look for carotid stenosis

Chronic Stroke Management

- Once the acute phase has passed, the patient is still at increased risk of having another stroke. We want to prevent another one from happening
  - This is called **secondary prevention**
- If cardiac embolism is the cause of the stroke, use warfarin (goal INR 2-3) or factor Xa/direct thrombin inhibitor (rivaroxaban, apixaban, dabigatran)
- If thrombotic stroke, use ASA 81 mg
- If thromboembolism from carotid stenosis, use ASA/dipyridamole combination

- If carotid stenosis is > 70% and symptomatic, perform carotid endarterectomy (CEA)

- Longterm, maintain normotension, healthful diet, normal blood sugar and cholesterol, active lifestyle with regular aerobic exercise, stop smoking, achieve normal BMI

- Prognosis: **most recovery in a stroke will occur within the first 3-6 months**
  - Motor, speech, swallowing, bowel, bladder

The Circle of Willis

- "Classic" anatomy, but not common anatomy

- Anterior and posterior (vertebrobasilar) circulation systems

- Let's draw it out and discuss common spots where things tend to go wrong

Cerebrovascular Territories

- **Anterior cerebral artery (ACA):** commands the leg muscles and executive function
  - Basically the medial surface of the brain in a sagittal view

- **Middle cerebral artery (MCA):** commands the face and upper extremity muscles, language, and spatial perception
  - Basically the outside convexity of the brain in a sagittal view as well as deeper until you reach the medial ACA territory

- **Posterior cerebral artery (PCA):** commands cerebellar and visual cortices

- Let's draw it out to make a little more sense of it

Cerebrospinal Fluid (CSF) Flow

- Choroid plexus (lateral ventricles) → foramina of Monro → third ventricle → cerebral aqueduct → fourth ventricle → foramen of Magendie → foramina of Luschka → subarachnoid space (brain, spinal cord)

- Let's draw it out to make more sense of it

Brainstem Anatomy

- The brainstem is supplied by the vertebrobasilar system (posterior circulation)

- **The brainstem rule of 4**
  - There are 4 cranial nerve nuclei per segment of brainstem (midbrain, pons, medulla)
  - There are 4 **m**idline structures that start with **M**
    - Motor pathway, medial lemniscus, medial longitudinal fasciculus, motor nuclei
  - There are 4 **s**ide structures that start with **S**
    - Spinothalamic pathway, spinocerebellar pathway, sensory nucleus of CN5, sympathetic

- ○ There are 4 motor nuclei that divide equally from 12
  - ■ CN 3, 4, 6, 12 (1 and 2 aren't really in the brainstem so we leave them out)
- Using these rules you can identify the precise location of the patient's stroke within the brainstem, using the signs and symptoms as latitude and longitude

ACA Stroke

- Contralateral leg weakness and numbness distal>proximal
- Incontinence
- If bilateral: bilateral symptoms and executive function, personality deficits

MCA Stroke

- Contralateral face, arm, hand weakness and numbness with either aphasia (left brain lesion) or contralateral hemineglect (right brain lesion)
- Usually due to a cardiac embolism
- Usually superior division MCA strokes lead to Broca aphasia (expressive aphasia) and contralateral upper limb weakness
- Usually inferior division MCA strokes lead to Wernicke aphasia (receptive aphasia) or contralateral hemineglect

Aphasia

- Practice the aphasia tree to get good at it
- Anomia: fluent, can comprehend, can repeat, cannot name things
- **Broca** aphasia: nonfluent, can comprehend, cannot repeat
- Transcortical motor: nonfluent, can comprehend, can repeat
- **Wernicke** aphasia: fluent, cannot comprehend, cannot repeat
- Transcortical sensory: fluent, cannot comprehend, can repeat
- Mixed transcortical: nonfluent, cannot comprehend, can repeat
- Conduction: fluent, can comprehend, cannot repeat
- **We will draw this out to make sense of it**

Aphasia Treatment

- Aphasia treatment largely is a "wait and see" endeavor
- Speech therapy plays a central role in challenging the patient to re-develop normal speech and thought patterns
- **Melodic intonation therapy** is useful for Broca aphasia

- By singing your speech, you recruit the right brain to help with speech production

PCA Stroke

- Supplies chiefly the visual cortex, cerebellum, and midbrain
- Thus, deficits are in vision, coordination, and brainstem findings
- Remember your vision pathway to localize the lesion
    - Contralateral homonymous hemianopia is a common buzzword
    - Lesions at the optic chiasm lead to bitemporal hemianopia
- Anton syndrome: bilateral visual cortex strokes, leading to cortical blindness and patient denial of the blindness

Lacunar Strokes

- These are often "pure" (pure motor or pure sensory)
- Posterior limb of internal capsule / corona radiata
    - Contralateral hemiplegia
    - Pure motor syndrome
- Thalamus
    - Contralateral numbness
    - Pure sensory syndrome
    - Their neuropathic pain becomes very difficult to treat
- Movement disorders (basal ganglia)
    - Contralateral hemiballismus: subthalamic nucleus
    - Contralateral hemichorea: caudate nucleus
- Dysarthria / Clumsy Hand Syndrome
    - Dysarthria and clumsy hand due to contralateral pontine lesion

Brainstem Strokes

- The following slides will talk about different brainstem stroke syndromes
- Note that in all of them, there is no mention of aphasia or cognitive deficits!
- These strokes are all below the brain, so there is no aphasia, cognitive deficits, or personality disorders

Wallenberg Syndrome

- AKA lateral medullary syndrome
- "Dr. Horner Wallenberg at the VA says don't PICA horse that can't eat"
- VA/PICA stroke, hoarse voice (CN 9 lesion), dysphagia (CN 10 lesion)

- Ipsilateral Horner syndrome (ptosis, miosis, anhidrosis)
- The PICA is a cerebellar artery after all, so the patient may fall *towards* the side of the lesion

Weber Syndrome

- "I'm paralyzed by 3 Webs!"
- Weber syndrome → contralateral hemiparesis, ipsilateral CN 3 palsy
- This is a medial midbrain lesion
- If it's the midbrain...it's probably the PCA that's the culprit

Medial Medullary Syndrome

- Medial in the medulla → CN 12 is found there
  - You lick your wounds → tongue deviates toward side of lesion
- Medial in the medulla → motor pathway is found there
  - Contralateral hemiparesis (corticospinal tract)
- Medial in the medulla → medial lemniscus is found there
  - Contralateral numbness

Locked-In Syndrome

- AKA basilar artery occlusion syndrome
- Basilar artery occlusion leads to **tetraplegia with spared ability to move the eyes vertically and blink**
- Reticular activating system (RAS) is spared, as it mainly originates in the midbrain
  - Thus, **patient is fully conscious**

Stroke Rehabilitation

- How we get patients better after a stroke is three major things
  - Time
  - Using what we've got
  - Using what we get back
- We teach patients strategies to communicate and increase their mobility, ability to perform ADLs, and independence
- Let's talk about some different theoretical methods of rehabbing these patients
- These are basically different ways to theoretically drive the neurologic recovery and neuroplasticity

Stroke Recovery Patterns

- Patients tend to follow certain recovery patterns when recovering from a stroke

- **Hemiparesis,** for example, follows several stages:
    - 1 = totally flaccid
    - 2 = spasticity, hyperreflexia, UE flexor synergy pattern, LE extensor synergy pattern
    - 3 = spasticity peaks; control over synergy patterns begins
    - 4 = spasticity decreases; control is maximized
    - 5 = complex voluntary movements
    - 6 = spasticity gone
    - 7 = normal

- Note that with improved voluntary control comes decreased spasticity

Bobath/Neurodevelopmental Technique

- Seeks to rehab the patient by eliminating all primitive reflexes and flexor synergy patterns
    - Primitive reflexes: Babinski, palmomental (stroke thenar eminence → chin twitch)

- Inhibit spastic tone with therapy and orthoses

- Do not allow the patient to use flexor synergy or extensor synergy patterns to perform a task

- The idea is that we do not want to reinforce these primitive pathways, or else the patient may "stay that way"

Brunnstrom Technique

- Brunnstrom = villain

- The opposite of NDT

- Brunnstrom says to "use what you've got"
    - Use the flexor and extensor synergies, as it's all we've got, and there's no guarantee anything else will come back
    - Synergies can be used for ADLs, mobility, muscle conditioning

- You originally developed this way as an infant, so it's not that abnormal to re-do it while hoping more function comes back

Rood Technique

- Use cutaneous stimuli to enhance motor control and activity, and reduce spasticity

- Stretching, heat/ice, stroking, pushing, tapping, vibrating, etc. are all used to help facilitate recovery

Proprioceptive Neuromuscular Facilitation (PNF)

- Challenge patient's proprioceptive abilities by performing diagonal movement patterns in their therapies
- We don't normally perform activities like robots; we use diagonal movements in our daily lives; thus, therapies should emphasize this
- **Mnemonic: it takes proprioception to be able to perform a diagonal movement with your eyes closed; thus, this is the PNF theory**

Constraint-Induced Movement Therapy (CIMT)

- Restrain the "good" arm and force the paretic arm to work
- Do not do this in hemineglect; it will not work
- **Patient must have at least 10 degrees of active wrist extension to attempt this**

Medical Complications of Stroke

- Patients with stroke are commonly left with impairments such as dysphagia, neurogenic bowel and bladder, spasticity, shoulder pathology, CRPS, etc.
- Let's discuss each of these to get a good understanding of what they are and how to manage them

Dysphagia

- Normal swallowing takes place in 4 phases
  - Oral preparatory phase
    - Voluntary
    - Prepare bolus for swallowing
    - Soft palate compresses downward to seal the oral cavity
  - Oral phase
    - Voluntary
    - Tongue and soft palate rise as tongue compresses bolus and sends it into the esophagus
    - Tongue moves posteriorly to deliver bolus to esophagus
  - Pharyngeal phase
    - Involuntary
    - Bolus is transferred from oral cavity to esophagus
    - **This is typically when aspiration happens**
  - Esophageal phase
    - Involuntary

Dysphagia

- In stroke patients, this motor program is impaired, and patients are at risk for aspiration, most notably in the pharyngeal phase of swallowing
- Many stroke patients are made NPO, or are given a modified diet
- Thin liquids are more difficult to manipulate for stroke patients, as the liquid moves fast and is difficult to control; thus, thicker liquids are ordered to prevent aspiration
- Pudding-thick liquids are the thickest and easiest to swallow
- Honey-thick liquids are medium thickness
- Nectar-thick liquids are mild thickness
- Thin liquids are normal
- The thicker the liquid, the more time your oropharyngeal muscles have to coordinate properly and allow for a safe swallow

Dysphagia

- Modified diets include:
- Dysphagia level 1: puree, requiring no chewing
- Dysphagia level 2: mechanically altered
- Dysphagia level 3: soft, requiring some chewing
- Regular diet
- Patients progress from 1 → 3, and potentially regular diet
- Bedside swallow study is performed by speech therapist to assess for signs/symptoms of aspiration with the selected thickness (including liquids)
    - Cough, wet voice, altered vocal quality
    - Sometimes "silent aspiration" occurs, in which the patient aspirates but has no signs or symptoms of this on a bedside swallow
- Modified barium swallow (MBS)
    - Gold standard for studying a patient's swallow and fully evaluating dysphagia

Dysphagia

- Fiberoptic endoscopic evaluation of swallowing (FEES)
    - Endoscopic direct visualization of swallowing action
    - May be limited by presence of scope

Dysphagia

- If patient is unsafe per bedside swallow or MBS, consider non-oral means of feeding
    - Nasogastric tube (NG/duotube)
    - Gastric tube (G-Tube) if prolonged (> 2 weeks of unsafe swallow)

- Compensatory strategies in the meantime include **chin tuck** (pushes larynx away from pharynx and constricts the posterior pharynx to squeeze the bolus through and into the esophagus) and **head rotation** (turn head toward the paretic side, closing off the paretic side and facilitating normal swallowing)
- Dysphagia in stroke has a favorable prognosis overall in terms of having some diet reintroduced into the patient's life

Neurogenic Bladder

- Neurogenic bladder, leading to incontinence, is common after stroke
- Impaired mobility, cognition, and communication also contribute to incontinence
- Typically this is an **upper motor neuron, spastic bladder**
  - The bladder fills with only a little volume, then the detrusor spastically contracts to empty the bladder, causing incontinence
- The best treatment is a timed voiding program with fluid intake regulation
- Consider UTI as an etiology
- Anticholinergic medications are occasionally used (oxybutynin, tolterodine) to calm the bladder down and promote storage, but these can have cognitive side effects which we would like to avoid in stroke patients
- Sometimes clean intermittent catheterization is used (see SCI section)

Neurogenic Bowel

- Bowel incontinence is also common after stroke, but the incontinence typically resolves within the first 2 weeks
- Generally we treat this with a timed bowel program, maintaining a regular diet and bowel medication schedule (PEG, senna, suppositories, fiber), and improving mobility to get to the toilet

Deep Vein Thrombosis (DVT)

- Common after strokes (impaired mobility and muscle contraction)
  - Virchow Triad: stasis, endothelial injury, hypercoagulability
- Doppler ultrasound is typically used, often as a pre-inpatient rehab screening test
- D-dimer is sensitive but not specific for DVT
- **Prophylaxis** with subcutaneous heparin (SQH) or low-molecular weight heparin (enoxaparin)
  - Frequently will also see SCDs and compression stockings
- **Treatment** with heparin drip or increased enoxaparin dosage (1 mg/kg BID)
- IVC filter can be placed if patient is at too great of a risk to bleed with chemoprophylaxis

Complex Regional Pain Syndrome (CRPS)

- AKA reflex sympathetic dystrophy (RSD), shoulder-hand syndrome
- Essentially this is sympathetically mediated pain due to an unknown etiology that results in an area of the body having increased neuropathic pain, hypersensitivity, and allodynia, all in conjunction with detectable skin and vasomotor changes over the affected area on the body
- CRPS Type 1 = the above symptoms without a known peripheral nerve injury
- CRPS Type 2 = the above symptoms within a known peripheral nerve distribution
- CRPS has 3 different stages. We will discuss these in the Pain Medicine section.

Post-Stroke Shoulder Pain

- Post-stroke shoulder pain is common, and can be due to CRPS, post-thalamic stroke pain syndrome, or true MSK shoulder pathology
  - Rotator cuff tear/impingement, bursitis, adhesive capsulitis (frozen shoulder), biceps tendonitis
  - See MSK Shoulder section for this discussion

- **Shoulder subluxation**
  - Common in stroke patients
  - The rotator cuff maintains the humeral head within the glenoid cavity (socket)
  - Thus, when the cuff is paretic/plegic, the humeral head falls out of the glenoid
  - There is a palpable gap or sulcus when palpating the humeral head and the acromion
  - We are not really sure if shoulder subluxation causes pain, or if our subluxation cuffs do anything to "improve" the shoulder or help with pain, but these are common treatments regardless

- **Adhesive capsulitis (frozen shoulder)**
  - See MSK Shoulder section for this discussion
  - Note: adhesive capsulitis in stroke can be harder to treat than "normal" frozen shoulder

Post-Stroke Spasticity

- We've already discussed how spasticity develops after a stroke
  - Flaccid → spasticity and synergy patterns → peak spasticity → more control over synergies correlating with decreased spasticity → more complex control and even lower spasticity →→ normal
- Often this pathway is halted at step 3 (peak spasticity), and the patient is left to live with their spastic tone interfering with their function and posing a risk for skin breakdown

- Spasticity is a velocity-dependent increase in muscle tone (resistance to passive movement)
- We commonly treat it with oral, intrathecal, or injection-based medications
- See Spasticity section within the SCI Section for a full discussion
  - See Pharmacology section for a full medication discussion

Risk Factors for Not Returning to Work

- Major risk factors include a prolonged inpatient rehab stay and aphasia (difficult for patient to maintain "carryover" of therapy instructions if they have aphasia)

Movement Disorders

- The intracranial structures responsible for movement disorders are often damaged in stroke patients as well
- Given the intracerebral nature of these disorders, we will discuss them here
- Movement disorders are named so because they result in **abnormal, involuntary movement patterns of a patient's head or limbs**
- Usually the **basal ganglia** or **cerebellum** is involved
- The basal ganglia is a complicated network of nuclei in the brain that coordinates and executes movement programs originating in the premotor and motor cortices
- The cerebellum controls ipsilateral balance and coordination of movements

Movement Disorders

- **Ataxia:** impaired coordination typically due to cerebellar lesions
  - Cerebellar ataxia: due to cerebellar lesion
  - Sensory ataxia: due to impaired proprioception and sensation in the limbs
  - Vestibular ataxia: often due to lesions of the vertebrobasilar system, leading to impaired balance
    - Often nausea, vomiting, vertigo are present
- **Choreoathetosis:** involuntary dance-like, snake-like writhing movements of the limb
- **Hemiballismus:** violent, "ballistic" flinging motions of the limb due to a contralateral subthalamic nucleus lesion
- **Akathisia:** motor restlessness
- **Tics:** voluntary muscle contractions or posturing due to an inner tension or itch that needs to be relieved

Movement Disorders

- **Tremors**

- Essential tremor: involuntary rhythmic motion while trying to maintain the position of a limb
    - Benign
    - Propranolol or alcohol improve symptoms
- Intention tremor: involuntary rhythmic motion while trying to perform a limb action
    - Cerebellar lesion
    - Weights on the limb can help to stabilize it
- Resting tremor: involuntary rhythmic motion while limb is at rest
    - Often due to Parkinson Disease
    - "Pill-rolling tremor"

Movement Disorders

- **Dystonia**
    - Involuntary, abnormal muscle contractions resulting in abnormal posturing
    - Can be genetic, antipsychotic-related, or from intracranial damage
    - Some patients have Dopa-Responsive Dystonia which responds to levodopa-carbidopa
    - Cervical dystonia has various postures associated with it:
        - Anterocollis: bilateral SCM
        - Retrocollis: bilateral splenius capitis, spinal erectors
        - Torticollis: contralateral sternocleidomastoid (SCM), ipsilateral splenius capitis and levator scapula
        - Laterocollis: ipsilateral splenius capitis, scalenes, levator scapula
    - Botulinum neurotoxin is very effective for treatment

Movement Disorders

- **Myoclonus**
    - Sudden involuntary muscle contractions
    - Positive myoclonus: involuntary contraction
    - Negative myoclonus: involuntary relaxation
    - Treat with anticonvulsants or neurotoxin injection

Movement Disorders

- **Restless Leg Syndrome**
    - An abnormal, very uncomfortable feeling of intense tension and urge to move the legs
    - Sometimes this is due to iron deficiency anemia and can improve with iron therapy
    - Often we don't know why the patient has this
    - Treat with levodopa-carbidopa, ropinirole, pramipexole

■ All are dopaminergic agents

Movement Disorders

● **Huntington Disease**

   ○ Autosomal dominant CAG repeats cause abnormal Huntingtin protein to accumulate and cause degeneration of the caudate nucleus in the basal ganglia

   ○ Choreoathetosis develops

   ○ Anticipation takes place (earlier and earlier onset in subsequent generations)

   ○ Suicide is common

   ○ Treatment is aimed at decreasing dopamine and increasing acetylcholine to help decrease movement

      ■ Antipsychotics

      ■ SSRIs for depression

Movement Disorders

● **Parkinson Disease**

   ○ Degeneration of the substantia nigra neurons leads to decreased dopamine in the nigrostriatal pathway → little to no movement

   ○ TRAP

      ■ Tremor (resting 3-5 Hz)

      ■ Rigidity (cogwheel)

      ■ Akinesia

      ■ Postural instability

   ○ Treatment is aimed at increasing dopamine and decreasing acetylcholine

      ■ Levodopa-carbidopa

      ■ Amantadine (increases endogenous release of dopamine)

      ■ Benztropine (anticholinergic)

      ■ MAO-B or COMT inhibitors (decrease dopamine breakdown)

      ■ Deep brain stimulation (DBS) in subthalamic nucleus

   ○ Swallow evaluation is important as the movement disorder may manifest as dysphagia

Movement Disorders

● **Ataxia**

   ○ Friedreich Ataxia

      ■ Autosomal recessive

      ■ Affects teenagers

      ■ Scoliosis, wheelchair dependence, HOCM

   ○ Ataxia-Telangiectasia

      ■ Ataxia with skin telangiectasias

Congratulations on finishing Chapter 2! Knowing this chapter well will serve you very deeply on rotations and exams regarding the vast majority of stroke rehabilitation and movement disorder clinical knowledge and decision-making.

Chapter 3: Traumatic Brain Injury (TBI)

Definition and Epidemiology of TBI

- Disruption of normal brain function due to a physical blow to the head
- Falls vs MVAs as leading cause of TBI
- Single, white, undereducated teenage male (teenage to 25 yo)
- Alcohol is usually involved
- Most TBIs are mild (GCS 13-15)
- If elderly, falls
- If pediatric, MVA

Acute Management of TBI

- ABCs, standard emergency protocol
- CPP = MAP - ICP
  - CPP = cerebral perfusion pressure (**keep above 60** mmHg)
  - MAP = mean arterial pressure
  - ICP = intracranial pressure (normal is <15)
- Monitor ICP with intraventricular ICP catheter for severe TBIs
  - Can also check with lumbar puncture (LP)

Acute Management - Lowering ICP

- How do you lower ICP? (thus, keeping CPP high)
  - Normal range is 2-5 (keep it under 20)
- Use drugs that lower the volume of fluid in the brain
  - Hypertonic solutions, diuretics (e.g. IV mannitol, acetazolamide)
- Forced hyperventilation for quick lowering of pressure (not longterm)
  - Decreased $PaCO_2$ causes cerebral vasoconstriction, lowering blood volume in the brain
- Hypothermia

Acute Management of TBI

- Head CT without contrast!
- Later on, get MRI to assess grade of DAI
- Frequent neuro exams
  - Pupillary responsiveness is important prognostic factor
- Emergency neurosurgery

- o Burr hole, craniotomy
- o Usually in cases where something is there that shouldn't be
- Impending uncal herniation
  - o Unilateral blown pupil = emergency surgery!

Primary vs Secondary Injury

- **Primary injury** = immediate concussive force of the impact causing disruptive shear forces, brain contusions, and DAI.
- Contusions (brain bruises) usually happen at the "horns" of the brain
  - o Prominent, protruding areas of the brain
  - o **Inferior frontal lobe, anterior temporal lobes**
  - o Come into play in diaschisis
- **Diaschisis** = "split across"
  - o Damage one area, and you just damaged a remote region that was connected to that area
  - o Recovery in area 2 parallels recovery of area 1
- **DAI** = diffuse axonal injury

DAI (Diffuse Axonal Injury)

- Axons in the brain are injured due to the concussive blast to the head, which shears the axons inside and leads to central white matter damage (because that's where axons are)
  - o This damage lights up on **diffusion-weighted MRI** (**D**AI → **D**iffusion-weighted MRI)
  - o White matter locations are the things in the middle:
    - Brain stem
    - Corpus callosum
    - "Central white matter"

Grading DAI

- DAI is graded 1-3 (MRI criteria)
  - o 3 is the worst
- 1 = no focal changes on MRI
- 2 = focal changes (e.g. central white matter)
- 3 = brainstem involvement

Secondary Injury

- All the detrimental biochemical cascades that happen after the primary injury
- Excitatory toxicity (glutamate!)

- - Massive neurotransmitter surge
  - The brain burns out
- **Brain swelling**
  - Can see on head CT as **decreased size of ventricles**
- **Brain edema**
  - Longstanding, due to **blood vessel damage that causes fluid to leak out into the brain** tissue, as well as cells not doing their jobs well anymore and **building up fluid within themselves**

Posturing

- A patient may take on a posture after a TBI. This can be decorticate or decerebrate
- **Decorticate** posture
  - Arms flexed, legs extended
  - Due to **lesions above the brainstem**
- **Decerebrate** posture
  - Arms extended, legs extended
  - Due to midbrain lesion
  - Worse prognosis due to **brainstem involvement**

Brain Bleeds

- These happen due to blunt force of the trauma, but are more likely as you age
- **Epidural** hematoma
- **Subdural** hematoma
- **Subarachnoid** hemorrhage
- Order a **noncontrast head CT** to see the bleed!

Epidural Hematoma (EDH)

- Strike the middle meningeal artery → EDH
- No midline shift (it's **above** the dura)
- Lucid interval...then downhill fast

Subdural Hematoma (SDH)

- Long, crescent-shaped opacity due to rupture of the thin bridging veins between the dura and arachnoid (**subdural**)
- Old age → brain atrophy → these veins get stretched and are more likely to snap/rupture
- **Acute** (immediate-onset)

- **Subacute** (1-3 weeks) (alcoholics)
- **Chronic** (longer than that)

Subarachnoid Hemorrhage (SAH)

- Usually from a ruptured AVM or berry aneurysm (usually Acomm or Pcomm)
- See blood in the subarachnoid space on head CT
- Give nimodipine x21 days to prevent cerebral vasospasm

Cranial Nerve Injuries

- Some common cranial nerves that are injured in TBIs are:
- **CN1:** it's #1, and as such it is the most often injured CN in TBIs
  - Altered smell and taste, lack of interest in eating, possibly weight loss due to this
- **CN2:** visual field deficits
- **CN7:** deficits in anterior ⅔ tongue taste, facial expression, salivation, tears
- **CN8:** hearing and balance loss.
  - If a patient with TBI is dizzy, though, it's probably just **BPPV**

Slight Detour...Brain Tumors

- Most common initial presentation of brain tumor is headaches with cognitive deficits
  - Order MRI with contrast
- After resection, patient may present like a TBI patient
- Can have nice functional gains at inpatient rehab
- **In kids**, cerebellar astrocytoma or medulloblastoma
  - #1 and #2 most common posterior fossa tumors
- **In adults,** glioblastoma multiforme (GBM)
- **If it's metastasis,** it's lung
- If they had whole-brain radiation, use steroids to reduce brain swelling

Ok...so that's all bad

- What **can** the brain do to help itself?
- 1. The brain is alive! Er...**plastic**.
  - Existing neurons can sprout new connections
  - Existing brain areas can be repurposed to perform the functions of a dead area
  - Totally unrelated areas can step up and perform a dead area's function
- 2. It has backups.

- Redundancy = if you damage one area, your brain has backup areas that can step in

Consciousness

- Basically the state of being awake and aware of one's self and surroundings
- The RAS regulates consciousness
- Consciousness has 4 states
    - Coma
    - Vegetative State (VS)
    - Minimally Conscious State (MCS)
    - Normal (emerged)
- You have a better prognosis each time you upgrade states

Coma

- Eyes closed
- **No** sleep/wake cycles on EEG
- **No** purposeful behavior or comprehension
- In short...you've got **nothing**

Vegetative State

- Eyes open
- **You DO have sleep/wake cycles on EEG**
- **No** localization of objects
- You DO have reflexive behaviors, but **you will NOT cross midline**
- **Persistent VS:** VS for over 1 month
- **Permanent VS:** VS for over 1 year after TBI, or over 3 months on nontraumatic BI
    - You get a little more leeway if you're a TBI

Minimally Conscious State

- Evidence of self or environmental awareness with purposeful behaviors and crossing the midline
- **Ok...so aren't you just...conscious?**
- Nope, it's all inconsistent, so you're **minimally** conscious

Normal/Emerged

- **Consistently** follow commands and communicate

Treatment for these DOCs

- DOC = disorder of consciousness

- The best treatment is supportive. Protect the patient and preserve what you can.

- You can try neurostimulation with drugs that increase dopamine in the brain
    - Amantadine: best studied, probably most commonly used
    - Methylphenidate
    - Modafinil (provigil)

Glasgow Coma Scale (GCS)

- GCS goes from 3-15 (15 is normal)

- **Mild TBI = concussion = GCS 13-15**

- **Moderate TBI** = GCS 9-12

- **Severe TBI = coma** = GCS 3-8

- You add up a patient's motor response (1-6), verbal response (1-5), and eye opening ability (1-4)

- The motor response has the highest value you can achieve in any category, so **motor response is the most important predictor of outcome in GCS**

Posttraumatic Amnesia (PTA)

- Just what it sounds like: you can't make memories of your daily events to remember what's going on around you in your daily life

- The sooner you get out of PTA, the better!
    - How do you know you're out?

- **GOAT!**
    - Galveston Orientation and Amnesia Test
    - Score 75 or higher for 2 straight days
    - Technically PTA is over once you've scored **75 or higher on the first** of these two passed tests

- Orientation Log
    - 25 or higher for 2 straight days

Glasgow Outcome Scale

- GOS = glasgow outcome scale
    - Scored 1-5. **Like GCS, you want to be high.**
    - 1 = dead
    - 2 = VS
    - 3 = conscious but dependent

- o   4 = independent but disabled
- o   5 = independent

Rancho Los Amigos

- Rancho is scored 1-8
- 1 = no response
- 2 = generalized response
- 3 = localized response
- 4 = confused agitated
- 5 = confused inappropriate
- 6 = confused appropriate
- 7 = automatic appropriate
- 8 = purposeful appropriate

Longterm Management of TBIs

- All doom and gloom...how do we manage these things?
  - o   Posttraumatic seizure (PTS) → a seizure after TBI → simple partial
  - o   Posttraumatic epilepsy (PTE) → recurrent seizures after TBI → AEDs
  - o   Posttraumatic hydrocephalus → increased pressure → relieve the pressure (VP shunt)
  - o   Dysautonomia/sympathetic storm → massive sympathetic output → propranolol
  - o   Agitation → reduce stimuli, let them burn off energy harmlessly
  - o   SIADH → too much ADH → restrict water
  - o   CSW → hypovolemic hyponatremia → IV fluids
  - o   DI → you have no ADH, so you pee out all your water → give them ADH

Posttraumatic Seizure (PTS)

- Having a seizure after a TBI, usually within the first 2 years
- Usually simple partial
- Immediate (0-1 day after TBI)
- Early (1-7 days)
- Late (over 7 days)
- Check a prolactin level if you suspect a seizure, as it will be increased
- EEG

Posttraumatic Epilepsy (PTE)

- Recurrent seizures after the first week, DUE TO THE TBI
- Risk factors for PTE? Having things in the brain that shouldn't be there
  - Foreign bodies (bullets, knife)
  - Blood (EDH/SDH/SAH/IPH)
  - Bony fracture
  - Abnormal neuronal discharge (early seizure)
- 1 week of AED prophylaxis, but continue it for 2 years if a late seizure occurs
- Levetiracetam (well tolerated), carbamazepine (hyponatremia, agranulocytosis), valproate (hepatotoxic - LFTs), phenytoin, phenobarbital

Dysautonomia / Sympathetic Storming

- Massive catecholamine surge that causes a huge sympathetic burst in the body, thus **hypertension, tachycardia, sweating, spasticity, fever**
- Occurs in spurts/paroxysms
- Manage with lipophilic beta blockers (**propranolol**), scheduled pain control (acetaminophen), dopamine agonists (bromocriptine, amantadine)
- Don't forget **infectious workup** if patient doesn't have a history of storming!

Posttraumatic Hydrocephalus (PTH)

- Usually due to subarachnoid hemorrhage
- Dilated ventricles with nausea/vomiting/headache/confusion
- Treat with VP shunt or serial lumbar punctures

Agitation

- "Agitation" means nothing!
- Ask what it means before reaching for the haldol
  - Physical? Verbal? Emotional? Just restless?
- Usually occurs in frontal lobe and temporal lobe lesions
- Agitation behavior scale (ABS)
  - < 21 is normal
  - > 34 is severe agitation

Treating Agitation

- Reduce stimuli
  - Lights/sounds/interactions/# people
- Let them burn off energy

- If physically aggressive and the above fails
  - Use antipsychotics/D2 blockers
  - Haloperidol can slow motor recovery
  - Quetiapine, olanzapine, ziprasidone, risperidone are popular
  - Watch for metabolic issues, **prolonged QT**
  - Lorazepam, propranolol, mood stabilizers, SSRIs can work

Electrolyte and Volume disorders

- Stem from pituitary dysfunction, and result in…
  - SIADH
  - CSW
  - DI

SIADH

- Syndrome of inappropriate ADH secretion = too much ADH!
- Too much ADH → too much water → **euvolemic hyponatremia**
  - **Normal HR and blood pressure**
- Caused directly by the brain trauma (TBI)
- Carbamazepine can also cause SIADH

Cerebral Salt Wasting (CSW)

- You lose salt → water follows → you've now lost salt **and** water → **hypovolemic hyponatremia**
- Tachycardia and low blood pressure (signs of hypovolemia)
- ADH is **appropriately elevated** here
- Both SIADH and CSW cause altered mental status (AMS)

Diabetes Insipidus

- You have no ADH → your body pees out all its water → you're THIRSTY
- Hypernatremia with dilute urine

Treating These Sodium/Water Disorders

- **SIADH** → restrict water
  - Use demeclocycline in resistant cases (it blocks ADH action in the kidney)
- **CSW** → IV fluids
- **DI** → they have no ADH, so just give them ADH (vasopressin/DDAVP)
- Patients often incontinent with these disorders

- ○   Timed bladder voids with frequent bladder emptying and training
- ○   May need to rule out UTI

Concussion (Mild TBI = GCS 13-15)

- Headache, sensory issues, psych issues, memory problems, sleep problems, tired all the time

- Brain trauma with LOC < 30min or PTA < 1 day or AMS or focal neuro deficits

- NOT mild if GCS < 13

- Concussions should recover within 1-3 months. If it doesn't you have **postconcussion syndrome**, which is having 3 of the above symptoms for 3 or more months with a demonstrated cognitive deficit, **and** this interferes with your daily life

What is the Protocol for Returning to Play?

- Essentially follows an NFL schedule (get you back on the field in 7 days)

- Progress to the next stage when asymptomatic at current stage for 1 day

- **Stage 1** = do nothing

- **Stage 2** = light cardio

- **Stage 3** = directional cardio (cardio + directional movement)

- **Stage 4** = sport-specific cardio (drills)

- **Stage 5** = full practice

- **Stage 6** = cleared to play NOW

Congratulations on finishing Chapter 3! The scales, numbers, and terminology of TBI may be new to you, but knowing these fundamentals will benefit you greatly in managing TBI patients and exam questions.

Chapter 4: Spinal Cord Injury (SCI), Spasticity, and Multiple Sclerosis

SCI Definition and Epidemiology

- Injury to the neural tissue within the spinal canal, resulting in variable weakness, sensory abnormalities, reflex changes, and autonomic dysfunction.

- Weakness, hyperreflexia, primitive reflexes (e.g. Babinski), neurogenic bowel and bladder, numbness/sensory changes

- Risk for certain conditions like spasticity, skin breakdown (pressure injuries), and autonomic dysreflexia

- On average it afflicts a single male in his 40s due to MVA in summertime

- Elderly are also common, often due to falls

- Incomplete tetraplegic > complete paraplegia = incomplete paraplegic > complete tetraplegic.

Spine and Spinal Cord Anatomy

- 7 cervical vertebrae

- 12 thoracic vertebrae

- 5 lumbar vertebrae

- 5 sacral vertebrae

- Central canal through which runs the spinal cord

- The spinal cord becomes the cauda equina around L1
    - The spinal cord is the conus medullaris at this level

- The cord is supplied by the **anterior spinal artery** (from VAs) for the anterior 2/3 of the cord, and posterior spinal arteries for the posterior cord

- The **Artery of Adamkiewicz** supplies the lower 2/3 of the cord

- Ischemia is more likely in the watershed region between these two blood supplies (lower thoracic region)

- Different tracts run through the spinal cord

Traumatic Ways to Injure the Spinal Cord

- Typically trauma (MVAs, falls) is the cause of SCI. Usually MVAs > falls.

- Spine fractures result and can damage the spinal cord via mechanical deformation of the cord

- The workup for spine fractures is typically with xrays, CT scan, and/or MRI

- **Most things in the cervical cord happen at the C5-C6 level**

- Let's talk about some of the bony injuries that can cause SCI

C1 Burst Fracture (Jefferson Fracture)

- This is due to high axial impact load at the top of the head, resulting in a burst fracture of the anterior or posterior arches of the C1 (Atlas) vertebra

- Typically there is no SCI with this, and it is stable

- Treatment: usually cervical brace (e.g. Halo), or surgery if unstable fracture

C2 Fractures

- **Dens (odontoid) fracture**

- Type 1: tip of dens fracture

- Type 2: fracture at base of odontoid

- Type 3: fracture at base of odontoid extending into C2 vertebra itself

- **Type 2 is most common and often requires surgery**

- The others usually do not require surgery

- **C2 Burst Fracture (Hangman Fracture)**

- Similar to C1 - fracture of the bony ring

- Due to rapid deceleration injury of the neck

- Treatment: cervical bracing vs. surgery if unstable

Cervical Compression/Hyperextension Fractures

- **Cervical compression fracture**

- Typically due to flexion and axial load, causing cervical VB fracture

- Anterior wedging of the VB occurs

- Disc or bony fragments can shoot into the spinal canal and injure the cord

- Treatment: cervical brace vs. surgical decompression

- **Hyperextension Injury**
  - Excessive hyperextension forces that usually result in a central cord syndrome
  - E.g elderly falling onto outstretched chin
  - Treatment: often can treat with cervical collar

Cervical Facet Joint Dislocations

- AKA "Jumped facets"

- Due to flexion +/- rotation

- The facet jumping narrows the spinal canal, compromising the cord and/or nerve roots

- o E.g. C6-C7 jumped facet may cause cervical myelopathy and/or C7 radiculopathy
- **Unilateral**
  - o C5-C6 level most common
  - o One side has a jumped facet while the other is normal
- **Bilateral**
  - o C5-C6 level most common
  - o Both sides (left and right) have jumped facets
- Treatment: surgical stabilization is often required

Thoracic and Lumbar Fractures

- **VB Compression or Burst Fracture**
  - o High mechanical axial forces crushing the VB, causing anterior wedging of the VB and sometimes retropulsed bony fragments into the spinal canal
- **Chance Fracture**
  - o Fracture that extends from the spinous process all the way through the bones and into the VB
  - o Due to trauma/falls
- Treatment: both are often neurologically stable and require only bracing
  - o Jewett or CASH brace to limit hyperflexion (see Prosthetics and Orthotics section)

Nontraumatic Ways to Injure the Spinal Cord

- **Anoxia:** often due to inadequate blood flow during vascular surgery
  - o E.g. aorta surgery requiring clamping of an aortic segment
- **Epidural abscess:** due to IVDA, immunocompromise, DM
- **Spinal cord tumor:** usually epidural (extradural) thoracic spine due to breast/prostate/lung mets
- **Radiation myelopathy:** prior history of radiation can lead to neuronal degeneration within the cord months/years later
- **Transverse myelitis:** inflammation of spinal cord due to unknown cause
- **Spinal stenosis:** spondylosis and arthritic changes in the spinal column can cause narrowing of the spinal canal, leading to cord compression and myelopathy

Types of SCI

- Complete vs. Incomplete
- Tetraplegia vs. Paraplegia
- Paresis vs. Plegia

- Complete: essentially no voluntary motor or sensory function below the level of the lesion

- Incomplete: there is some degree of motor and/or sensory function below the level of the lesion

- **Tetraplegia:** cervical spinal cord injury resulting in weakness and/or sensory abnormalities in all 4 limbs

- **Paraplegia:** thoracic or lumbosacral spinal cord injury resulting in weakness and/or sensory abnormalities in the lower limbs

Features of an SCI Patient

- **Upper motor neuron injury (UMN)** - true "cord" injury
  - Weakness in myotomes at and below level of injury
  - Hyperreflexia/clonus, +Babinski, +Hoffman
  - Spasticity
  - Impaired light touch or pinprick sensation in injured dermatomes
  - Spastic bladder (UMN bladder, overactive bladder, failure to store)
  - Lower baseline blood pressure

- **Lower motor neuron injury (LMN)** - more of a nerve root/axon injury within the central canal
  - Weakness and atrophy in myotomes at and below level of injury
  - Hyporeflexia/areflexia
  - Impaired light touch or pinprick sensation in injured dermatomes
  - Hypoactive bladder (LMN bladder, underactive bladder, failure to empty)

The ASIA Exam

- A systematic way to define the extent of a patient's SCI
  - Complete vs. incomplete, tetra vs. para, is there any motor or sensory function spared below the level of the injury?

- Performed in 3 stages
  - Motor testing (myotome scan)
  - Sensory testing (light touch and pinprick in all dermatomes)
  - Rectal tone and sensation

ASIA Motor Exam

- This is a myotome scan including C5-T1 and L2-S1
- Strength grading from 0-5 (2-5 must be through full ROM!)
- C5 = elbow flexors (biceps brachii)
- C6 = wrist extensors (ECRL/ECRB)

- C7 = elbow extensors (triceps)
- C8 = finger flexors (FDP)
- T1 = pinky abductors (ADM)
- L2 = hip flexors (iliopsoas)
- L3 = knee extensors (quadriceps)
- L4 = dorsiflexors (tibialis anterior)
- L5 = big toe extensors (EHL)
- S1 = plantarflexors (gastrocnemius)

ASIA Sensory Exam

- You will use a fluffy cotton swab and a safety pin to test light touch and pinprick, respectively
  - Light touch tests the dorsal columns
  - Pinprick tests the spinothalamic tracts
- Patient must commit to a response
  - 0 = no sensation whatsoever
  - 1 = feel it, but it is different when compared to face sensation
  - 2 = normal; feels the same as it does on the face

ASIA Rectal Exam

- Test sensory levels S3-S5 as you did the other dermatomes
- Test rectal wall sensation by asking if the patient can feel which direction your finger is pointing in and guess correctly
- Test rectal motor function by asking patient to squeeze down on your finger

ASIA Grading

- Gather motor levels, sensory levels, neurologic level of injury (NLI)
- There are 2 motor levels and 2 sensory levels (1 for each side)
- Motor level = the most distal myotome that is at least 3/5 in strength AND all myotomes above it are normal 5/5
- Sensory level = the most distal dermatome that is 2/2 AND all dermatomes above it are 2/2
- NLI = the worst level out of all of those 4 above
- Once you have your NLI, you decide whether the injury is ASIA A, ASIA B, ASIA C, ASIA D, or ASIA E
- ASIA A is a complete injury

- ASIA B-E are all incomplete

ASIA Grading

- ASIA A = complete injury. No motor or sensory function at all below the NLI
    - NOON sign on the ASIA sheet
    - You may have zones of partial preservation (ZPP), which are just spotty, patchy areas below the NLI where motor or sensory function is somewhat intact
- ASIA B = some sensory sparing below the NLI with no motor function more than 3 levels below each **motor level (not NLI)** on each side
    - No NOON sign is present by definition
    - S4-S5 or deep anal sensation is intact
- ASIA C = there is voluntary anal contraction OR some motor function is preserved below the NLI
- ASIA D = there is voluntary anal contraction AND some motor function is preserved below the NLI AND >50% of these muscles are 3/5 or better
- ASIA E = had a previous ASIA-documented injury and is now normal

ASIA Quick-Grading

- Basically, look at your sheet, and check for a NOON sign
    - If NOON sign → ASIA A, then list any ZPPs
- Is there voluntary anal contraction?
    - If yes, automatically a C or D
    - If no, check for motor function more than 3 levels below the motor level on either side
        - If there is, automatically a C or D
    - If no VAC or motor function, no NOON sign → ASIA B
- Of the muscles below the NLI, are >50% of them 3/5 strength or better?
    - If no → ASIA C
    - If yes → ASIA D
- Is everything normal on the exam?
    - If yes → ASIA E

Anterior Cord Syndrome

- Loss of blood supply from the ASA or Artery of Adamkiewicz, resulting in injury to the anterior 2/3 of the spinal cord (this leaves only the dorsal columns intact)
- Anterior cord syndrome can also occur due to retropulsed disc/bone fragments, trauma
- Bilateral: weakness, impaired pain and temperature sensation, UMN bowel and bladder dysfunction, impaired coordination

Posterior Cord Syndrome

- Rare
- Injury to the dorsal columns of the spinal cord, resulting in bilateral impaired light touch, pressure, proprioception at and below the level of injury
- These patients ambulate very poorly

Central Cord Syndrome

- Usually an elderly fall + hyperextension injury (landing on the outstretched chin), resulting in injury to the central cord elements
- This is the most common incomplete SCI
- UE > LE, distal > proximal weakness
  - Essentially, hand weakness more so than any other muscles
  - If anything else is injured, it will recover faster than the hands
- Possible UMN bowel/bladder and sensory dysfunction
- Being young <50 is better prognosis

Brown-Sequard Syndrome

- Essentially a cord hemisection due to trauma (knife, bullet)
- Ipsilateral loss of motor function, coordination, and light touch/proprioception
- Contralateral loss of pain/temperature below level of injury

Conus Medullaris Syndrome

- Conus medullaris is the terminal cord around the L1 level
- Injury due to trauma, burst fracture, tumor
- Symmetric, with variable bowel/bladder dysfunction, often normal motor function
  - Conus is the launchpad for S1-S5 roots, so you may see calf and rectal tone weakness
  - L1-L5 roots have already come off the cord at this point, so they should be unaffected
- Hyperreflexia is a possibility, especially in S1 root
- EMG not informative (UMN injury)

Cauda Equina Syndrome

- LMN injury to the L1-S5 roots (axons) of the cauda equina
  - "What you hit is what you hit"

- Due to trauma, burst fracture, tumor

- Asymmetric, variable myotome weakness and dermatome sensory loss

- Areflexic, LMN bowel and bladder

- Hyporeflexia/areflexia

- EMG can offer prognosis

Gait Prognosis in SCI

- C1-T9 = nonambulatory

- T10-L2 = ambulate with KAFOs, forearm crutches

- L3-S5 = ambulate with KAFOs/AFOs, forearm crutches vs. cane

Medical Complications of SCI

- SCI results in impairments in bowel and bladder function, abnormal muscle tone (spasticity), risk of skin breakdown, impaired autonomic regulation (sweating, blood pressure, HR, temperature regulation), impaired respiration, autonomic dysreflexia

- Acutely we see spinal shock

Spinal Shock

- In acute SCI, we see immediate absence/delay of all spinal reflex activity below the level of injury, including autonomics (sweating, vasomotor control)

- Essentially, think of everything as flaccid and just "sitting there"

- This lasts for 24 hours, then we see return of reflexes/function

- Babinski: delayed curling of the toes compared to normal
    - This is the first reflex to return

- Anal wink: stimulate perianal region and see reflexive anal contraction

- Bulbocavernosus: squeeze tip of penis or clitoris and see anal contraction

- If none of these comes back, consider LMN injuries

Autonomic Dysreflexia

- Injuries to the cord at T6 or above can put a patient at risk for AD

- Autonomic dysreflexia = "autonomic sixreflexia"

- Essentially, a noxious stimulus causes a massive reflex sympathetic surge that goes unregulated, resulting in bradycardia and HTN
    - Noxious stimulus = full bladder, pressure ulcer, skin wound, tight clothing, full bowel, ingrown toenail, visceral organ damage; a huge variety of causes exists
    - The pathway for descending sympathetic control is blocked by the SCI

- ○ Bradycardia is due to local vasoconstriction
- ○ This vasoconstriction causes the heart to try to compensate by slowing down (bradycardia via the intact vagus nerve)
- Usually at risk since 2 weeks after injury; complete are SCIs most at risk
- Headache, sweating above level of SCI, HTN (20 mm Hg above baseline), bradycardia → can lead to MI, stroke, SAH, seizures

Autonomic Dysreflexia Treatment

- Sit patient up, loosen clothing, cath bladder, check skin, evacuate bowels
- If not effective and SBP > 150
  - ○ Nifedipine 10 mg
  - ○ Clonidine 0.3 mg
  - ○ Nitroglycerin topical onto the chest (wear gloves!), then wipe away once noxious stimulus is removed

Impaired Temperature Regulation

- SCIs at T8 or above are at risk for impaired temperature regulation
- Use layers PRN for comfort

Orthostatic Hypotension

- SCI impairs ability to sympathetically constrict blood vessels to maintain bp
- Thus, if suddenly going from supine to sitting upright, patient pools all the blood in their legs since they can't constrict vessels to squeeze it back up to their brain
- Thus, they pass out - syncope, tachycardia
- Lie them flat or in Trendelenburg position with compression garments and abdominal binder applied
- Consider increased fluids +/- salt tabs, and midodrine +/- fludrocortisone for more vasoconstriction and bp support chronically

Pressure Injuries

- Breakdown of the skin +/- muscle, tendon, fat, bone exposure due to excessive longterm pressure or shear forces over an area of skin
  - ○ Too much pressure without shifting around means blood cannot flow to that area of skin
    - ■ Capillary ischemia to that area of skin if pressure is > 70 mmHg
- Sacrum is most common site
- In children, occiput is most common site
- Bony prominences are most at risk (above, + greater trochanters, ischia, heels)

- Prevent pressure ulcers by turning patient Q2H, repositioning Q20min otherwise, and having a nice pressure-relieving wheelchair seat cushion with tilt-in-space mechanism

Pressure Injuries

- <u>NPUAP Pressure Injury Staging</u>
- 1 = nonblanchable erythema (red skin that stays red when you press on it)
- 2 = skin breakdown extends into the dermis
- 3 = through the dermis with subQ fat exposed
- 4 = muscle, tendon, or bone is exposed
- Deep tissue injury = purple, intact skin, but the wound bed cannot be visualized
- Unstageable = really a stage 3 or 4, but you can't tell because there is so much slough/debris
- Once a stage X, always a stage X, no matter if it is now fully healed

Pressure Injuries

- Treatment
  - Relieve pressure as already discussed
  - Stage 1 and 2 = above; if it's wet, dry it; if it's dry, wet it
  - Stage 3 and 4 = debridement of dead tissue, irrigation, wound vac, skin flap
- All require good nutrition, vitamin C, zinc, copper, protein

Neurogenic Bladder

- **Normal bladder function**
- Frontal lobe primary motor cortex allows voluntary contraction/relaxation of external urethral sphincter
- Frontal lobe inhibits the sacral micturition center (which is parasympathetic)
- Pontine micturition center coordinates bladder (detrusor) contracting with internal urethral sphincter relaxing
- Sacral micturition center allows parasympathetic micturition action
  - **P**arasympathetics **P**ee **P**elvic

Neurogenic Bladder

- Voluntary nerve: pudendal nerve S2-S4
  - Voluntary contraction of external urethral sphincter (storage)
- Parasympathetic nerve: pelvic nerve S2-S4
  - **P**arasympathetics **P**ee **P**elvic

- Activate muscarinic ACh receptors in bladder wall which cause detrusor contraction (emptying) (using ACh)
- Sympathetic nerve: hypogastric nerve T11-L2
  - **Hypo**gastric nerve makes your bladder as big as a **hippo**
  - Activate α-1 and β-2 receptors to allow bladder storage (using norepinephrine)
  - α-1 in internal urethral sphincter causes sphincter contraction (storage)
  - β-2 in bladder wall causes relaxation of detrusor (storage)

Neurogenic Bladder

- In SCI, you may have UMN/spastic bladder or LMN/flaccid bladder, but most commonly we see DSD (detrusor-sphincter-dyssynergia)
- UMN bladder
  - Spastic; fails to store; fills up with a tiny amount of urine and then spastically clamps down using an overactive detrusor (loss of descending inhibition to the sacral micturition center from frontal lobe and pontine micturition center)
  - High vesicular (bladder) pressures result
  - Urine jets out (incontinence)
- LMN bladder
  - Flaccid; fails to actually empty; fills up with a huge amount of urine and still does not contract
  - Sacral micturition center control is blocked → cannot urinate
  - Urine leaks out (overflow incontinence)

Neurogenic Bladder

- DSD (detrusor-sphincter-dyssynergia)
  - Most common bladder pathology in SCI
  - Lesion somewhere between the brain and bladder (e.g. spinal cord)
  - The coordination between contracting the bladder and relaxing the sphincters is not there
  - Thus, spastic bladder results with impaired coordination of the sphincters, and high vesicular pressures as a result
  - Vesicoureteral reflux (VUR) is a complication

Neurogenic Bladder

- Urodynamic studies
  - Used to evaluate what exactly the bladder is doing when it fills and tries to void
  - We can detect UMN/LMN/DSD bladders and characterize them with this
  - We can detect VUR
- Treatment of neurogenic bladder

- Clean intermittent catheterization (CIC) Q4-6 hours
    - Keep cath volumes < 500 cc
- Anticholinergic bladder medications to prevent detrusor contraction and thus promote continence
    - Oxybutynin, tolterodine, mirabegron
    - Side effects: constipation, dry mouth
- Alpha blockers to relax internal urethral sphincter and promote proper bladder emptying
    - Tamsulosin (can decrease bp)
- Bladder wall botulinum toxin
- Sphincterotomy surgery if refractory to the above

Neurogenic Bowel

- Normally the bowel is controlled by parasympathetic and sympathetic systems, which control the enteric nervous system, which has myenteric (Auerbach) and submucosal (Meissner) plexuses
    - **My**enteric has **my** (myo) in it, thus it is the motor plexus
    - **S**ubmucosal is **s**ensory plexus
    - These coordinate the bowel peristalsis
- Parasympathetic action is to digest, perform peristalsis, move things along
    - Vagus and pelvic nerves
- Sympathetic action is to store (bowel de-motility and internal anal sphincter contraction), and shunt blood away from the bowel
    - Hypogastric nerve
- Somatic nervous system allows voluntary control of external anal sphincter
    - Pudendal nerve

Neurogenic Bowel

- Normally stool fills the rectal vault, and this bowel wall distension sends signals to the pontine defecation center which then coordinates sphincter relaxation and propulsion of stool bolus out of the anus
- In UMN/spastic bowel
    - PS and S control of bowel are blocked; thus we rely on myenteric and submucosal reflex activity with the spinal cord
    - Food can still be moved along, but the internal and external anal sphincters are spastic and tight
- In LMN/flaccid bowel
    - Myenteric and submucosal plexuses push stool along, but because this is a LMN injury, reflex activity cannot aid in this and cause defecation
    - Trickier situation, harder to have consistent bowel movements

Neurogenic Bowel

- Treatment involves taking advantage of reflexes and medications
- Gastrocolic reflex: presence of food in stomach causes reflex defecation
  - Sit patient on commode 15-60 minutes after meal to take advantage of this
- Rectocolic reflex: rectal distension (by stool or by finger) causes reflex defecation
  - Digital stimulation is part of most bowel programs
- Note: these reflexes are also present in normal healthy patients
- Medications
  - Docusate: softens stool by pulling fluid into the gut lumen, makes it easier to move along
    - 100mg BID
  - Senna: irritates bowel wall and stimulates it to contract and move stool along (peristalsis)
    - 2 tablets 8 hours before targeted BM
  - Polyethylene glycol: osmotic agent that pulls water into gut lumen to push things along
    - 1 packet daily
  - Bisacodyl: rectal suppository that irritates the rectal wall and causes contraction → defecation

Neurogenic Bowel

- Perform timed bowel program every day at the same time to facilitate regular BMs
- Supplement with enemas if needed
- Supplementing with fiber can help bulk up stool
  - Especially useful for LMN bowel in which manual stool removal is often needed
- Commode is best, but side-lying is ok

Sexual Dysfunction in SCI

- **Females**
  - **Normal menstruation returns within several months after SCI, thus fertility is unaffected**
  - Normal sexual function involves genital stimulation traveling through pudendal nerve S2-S4, and traveling back down through parasympathetic pelvic nerve which causes mucus secretion and lubrication along with muscular changes
  - Females often have decreased sexual desire after SCI coinciding with poor psychological state
- **Males**

- ○ Poor semen quality and impaired erections cause **decreased male fertility after SCI**
- ○ Normally erections occur via psychogenic stimuli (from brain) and tactile stimuli sending afferent signals to spinal cord and back down parasympathetic fibers that cause dilation of the corpus cavernosum and increased blood flow to the penis
- ○ Ejaculation is via sympathetic (hypogastric nerve) fibers
- ○ **P**oint and **S**hoot → **p**arasympathetic and **s**ympathetic actions on the penis
- ○ **Treatment:** sildenafil (phosphodiesterase inhibitor), vacuums, implants, penile injections; electroejaculation assistance, sperm extraction

Urinary Tract Infections (UTIs)

- Most SCI patients are colonized with bacteria, thus if they are asymptomatic, do not treat the urinalysis (UA) with antibiotics
- Only treat if symptomatic (fever, chills, increased spasticity), >10 WBC in urine, and >100,000 bacteria on UA
  - ○ Essentially, treat if there is a clear UTI on UA with clear symptoms caused by it
- You may treat the UA if patient is asymptomatic but they are about to have a bladder study, existing bladder pathology such as VUR, or they are growing urease-producing bugs

Hypercalcemia/Hypercalciuria

- Stones, bones, groans in weeks following SCI
- Immobilization and lack of normal weight-bearing causes hypercalcemic state
- **Treatment:** IV fluids (normal saline), therapy, weight-bearing, bisphosphonates

Osteoporosis and Fractures

- Less weight-bearing in SCI patients means less bone mass
- Risk of fractures increases
- Distal femur fracture is common
  - ○ Surgery vs. splinting/casting depending on degree of osteoporosis as determined by orthopedic surgeon

Pulmonary Insufficiency in SCI

- <u>Normal lung function</u>
- Inspiration
  - ○ Diaphragm contracts, thus sucking air into the chest cavity via the pull of negative pressure
    - ■ If breathing hard, external intercostals, scalenes, SCMs will help to expand ribcage

- Expiration
  - Mostly a passive process
  - Diaphragm relaxes, and air is passively pushed out of the chest cavity
    - If breathing hard, internal intercostals and abdominals can help expel air

Pulmonary Insufficiency in SCI

- <u>Lung volumes</u>
- Total lung capacity (TLC)
  - Total volume of air in the lungs at maximal inspiration
- Residual volume (RV)
  - The volume of air remaining in the lungs after a maximal expiration
- Vital capacity (VC)
  - The volume of air exhaled after maximal inspiration
- Forced expiratory volume in 1 second (FEV1)
  - The volume of air exhaled using maximal effort over the course of 1 second
- Forced vital capacity (FVC)
  - The volume of air exhaled during the FEV study (which overall lasts longer than 1 second)
- In SCI, you see a restrictive lung pattern
  - All lung volumes decrease, except RV

Pulmonary Insufficiency in SCI

- Cervical SCIs are most at risk for pulmonary insufficiency
  - The muscles of inspiration and expiration become nonfunctional
- The diaphragm is innervated by the phrenic nerve
  - C3,C4,C5 keep the diaphragm alive
- In C3 and C4 SCIs especially, the phrenic nuclei are damaged, causing potential inability to voluntarily inhale using the diaphragm
  - We use ventilators in these patients to keep them breathing
- In lower cervical injuries, we worry about abdominal and intercostal muscle paralysis
  - Inability to forcefully exhale and cough
  - Inability to use accessory muscles of inspiration and expiration
- Thoracic injuries cause varying degrees of abdominal and intercostal weakness

Pulmonary Insufficiency in SCI

- EMG of the diaphragm is useful to evaluate if the phrenic nerves and nuclei are intact

- ○ If intact and the lung function is not too impaired, we can implant a phrenic nerve or diaphragmatic pacer and use this to contract the diaphragm and inhale normally
- ○ If not intact, then we know we cannot do this
- Ultimately, SCI patients are most commonly left with a **restrictive lung pattern**
  - ○ All lung volumes decrease except residual volume
- Manage these patients with incentive spirometer, cough assist, coughalator (mechanical cough assist), suctioning, glossopharyngeal breathing

DVT/PE in SCI

- Virchow triad puts SCI patients at risk
  - ○ Stasis, endothelial injury, hypercoagulable state
- Warm, swollen limb
- **Workup:** doppler US, venogram
- Prophylaxis: **SQH or LMWH** until discharge (incomplete SCI) or for 8-12 weeks (complete SCI), SCDs, compression garments
- **Treatment:** heparin drip, LMWH 1 mg/kg BID, warfarin, rivaroxaban/apixaban/dabigatran
- DVT can cause pulmonary embolism (PE)
  - ○ Decreased O2 sats, tachypnea, chest pain, +D dimer,
  - ○ **Workup:** wedge-shaped opacity on xray, VQ scan, **helical CT scan with pulmonary arteriogram**
  - ○ **Treatment** = anticoagulation as above, embolectomy
- Consider PE prophylaxis with IVC filter if at too much risk for bleeding with AC

Causes of Death in SCI

- Acute = pulmonary embolism
- Chronic = pneumonia

Nociceptive and Neuropathic Pain in SCI

- **Nociceptive Pain**
  - ○ Often this is shoulder pain due to overuse of the GHJ (manual WC propulsion)
  - ○ Shoulder OA is common along with rotator cuff abnormalities, bursitis
  - ○ Treat as you would other patients with these disorders (RICE, NSAIDs, PT, injections)

- **Neuropathic Pain**
  - ○ Very common in SCI below the level of the injury
  - ○ Burning, tingling, electric, shooting pain

- Pregabalin is FDA approved
- We also use gabapentin, duloxetine, venlafaxine, anticonvulsants, topical lidocaine, topical capsaicin, topical diclofenac

Syringomyelia

- Insidious onset of ascending loss of reflexes, burning pain worse with sitting or valsalva, possible new myelopathy symptoms due to cystic cavitation of the central spinal cord that causes compression of the spinal cord
- New, progressive pain after an SCI → consider syringomyelia
- **Workup:** MRI with contrast
- **Treatment:** monitor with MRI and NSGY consult, avoid valsalva, neuropathic pain medications, shunting

Psychiatric Disease in SCI

- Depression is very common with increased risk of suicide in SCI patients
- Suicide is most common in paraplegics
- Treat with counseling, SSRIs, SNRIs

Surgical Interventions in SCI

- Tendon transfers
  - Must have 4 or 5 strength in the tendon being transferred since you usually lose a grade postsurgery
  - Transfer a functional level muscle to a nonfunctional level
    - E.g. C5 tetraplegia → transfer BR to ECRB to allow wrist extension
- Nerve grafting
  - Move functional healthy nerve to paralyzed muscle to allow it to grow into and reinnervate that muscle

Spasticity

- Spasticity = *velocity-dependent* resistance of a muscle to passive stretch
- Due to UMN lesion and thus the loss of descending inhibition upon the spinal cord and muscle reflex arc
  - SCI, TBI, stroke, MS
- Modified Ashworth Scale (MAS)
  - 0 = no spasticity (muscle is loosey-goosey throughout all ROM no matter how fast you move it)
  - 1 = catch and release at end range
  - 1+ = limb is easily ranged, but there is a catch and resistance to movement for **under** half of the ROM

- 2 = limb is easily ranged, but there is a catch and resistance to movement for **over** half of the ROM
- 3 = limb is difficult to range
- 4 = limb is rigid and will not move

Spasticity

- Spasticity can cause impaired ADLs (dressing, bathing, ambulation, etc.), skin breakdown (can't clean what you can't reach), pain, HO
- Spasticity can also aid function (utilize muscle tone to transfer surfaces), maintain muscle mass, and serve as a sentinel for infection (e.g. UTIs)
- We treat spasticity with PT, OT (involving lots of stretching and bracing), and medications
  - 4 FDA-approved medications for spasticity include baclofen, diazepam, tizanidine, and dantrolene

Spasticity

- **Baclofen** = centrally acting $GABA_B$ agonist
  - $GABA_A$ = binding here increases presynaptic Cl^- influx into the neuron
  - $GABA_{B1}$ = binding here inhibits presynaptic Ca^{2+} influx into the neuron
  - $GABA_{B2}$ = binding here increases postsynaptic K^+ conductance out of the neuron
    - All of these actions inhibit synaptic transmission and the firing of neurons
    - If you can't fire neurons, you can't fire muscles to make them contract
    - "CLACK"
      - Chloride, Calcium, Potassium
      - Cl, Ca, K
  - Dose: usually start 5 mg QHS, titrating up to 20-30 mg TID
  - Side effects: sedation, respiratory depression, lower seizure threshold
  - Withdrawal risk: "itchy, bitchy, and twitchy"
  - Clearance: renally cleared, so use lower doses in patients with CKD or select another agent

Spasticity

- **Diazepam** = centrally acting $GABA_A$ agonist (Cl^- channel activator)
  - CLACK!
- Dose: 2-10 mg TID
- Side effects: sedation, respiratory depression
- Withdrawal risk: seizures

- Clearance: hepatically cleared, so use caution with liver disease

Spasticity

- **Tizanidine** = centrally acting α_2 agonist (as is clonidine) which inhibits the spinal reflex arc
- Dose: usually start 2 mg QHS, then increase up to 12 mg TID (36 mg/day)
- Side effects: sedation, respiratory depression, lower seizure threshold
- Withdrawal: HTN, tachycardia, anxiety, worsened spasticity
- Clearance: hepatically cleared, so **check LFTs prior to dosing,** and monitor 1x per week for several weeks to ensure stability before spreading LFTs out over time

Spasticity

- **Dantrolene** = peripherally acting, binds to the ryanodine receptor on the sarcoplasmic reticulum in muscle cells, which then inhibits the influx of Ca^{2+} from the sarcoplasmic reticulum into the cell
    - No Ca^{2+} means the muscle can't contract
- Dosing: start 25 mg BID, titrating up to 400 mg/day (BID or TID dosing)
- Side effects: sedation, weakness
- Withdrawal: worsened spasticity
- Clearance: hepatically cleared, so **check LFTs prior to dosing,** and monitor 1x per week for several weeks to ensure stability before spreading LFTs out over time

Spasticity

- Which medication do I pick?
- SCI, MS: typically baclofen is the go-to, followed by tizanidine, due to familiarity and data in these populations
- Stroke, TBI: we often also use baclofen in these populations, but often we will instead prefer dantrolene first due to its peripheral action and theoretically less cognitively altering nature
- Diazepam is not as routinely used by physiatrists for spasticity compared to the other three medications

Spasticity

- Sometimes patients max out on oral medications (lack of efficacy, or too much sedation usually are the culprits)
- At this point we need to consider what else we can do for them
    - Intrathecal baclofen pump
    - Botulinum toxin injections

Spasticity

- **Intrathecal baclofen pump**
  - Works by surgically placing a pump reservoir into the patient's subcutaneous abdomen, with a catheter snaking out from the pump and working its way through the body and up into the intrathecal space of the spinal canal
    - The reservoir holds the baclofen medication
    - The catheter squirts that baclofen right into the CSF over the spinal cord
  - The benefit is that because the medication is squirted directly on top of the spinal cord, we can use doses in the pump that are far, far lower than oral doses, which means fewer side effects for the patient
  - Doses can be a simple continuous infusion of baclofen vs. squirting out boluses of baclofen at predefined intervals throughout the day and night

Spasticity

- Prior to pump implantation, patient must successfully respond via MAS tone reduction to a baclofen pump trial, in which a temporary catheter is placed into the intrathecal space, and doses of 50-100 mcg are administered
- Pumps have alarms that tell the patient when the medication is low, and when the medication is out
  - Withdrawal: "itchy, bitchy, and twitchy"
  - Supplement oral baclofen in this case if the patient is withdrawing
  - Usually pumps don't fail - people fail
- Pumps need to be refilled every 1-5 months

Spasticity

- **Botulinum toxin injections**
  - Botulinum neurotoxins inhibit the presynaptic syntaxin, synaptobrevin, and SNAP-25 proteins which are necessary to release neurotransmitters (Ach) into the synapse
  - By cleaving these proteins, the toxin prevents neurotransmitter (ACh) from being released
    - This is called chemodenervation
  - Thus, neurons can't fire, muscles can't contract, and you are paralyzed
  - By focally injecting this into select muscles, we can locally paralyze individual muscles, such as those that are too spastic
  - Black box warning of distant toxin spread, which may cause dysphagia, respiratory depression, so use with caution with existing motor neuron disease such as ALS
  - "3 days, 3 weeks, 3 months" (onset, peak, duration of action)

- Botulinum toxin is especially useful if you want to avoid systemic medications with systemic side effects

Multiple Sclerosis (MS)

- Autoimmune disease in which demyelinating plaques develop in the brain or spinal cord (CNS), causing UMN syndrome, bowel/bladder dysfunction, gait dysfunction, and psychiatric disturbances
  - Most commonly have pain, central fatigue, bowel/bladder dysfunction
- Oligodendrocytes make myelin in the CNS
  - They and their myelin become destroyed
- Patient is usually a white female in more northern latitudes
- There are 6 major types of MS

Multiple Sclerosis

- Relapsing-Remitting MS
  - Most common
  - Exacerbations followed by remissions
  - Generally patients have good return of function without severe disability
- Benign MS
  - Mild with mild/no disability, and complete remissions
- Primary Progressive MS
  - Does not have many remissions; just progresses steadily onward until patient dies with disability
- Malignant MS
  - Very severe, quick progression to disability and death

Multiple Sclerosis

- Good prognosis if...
  - Optic neuritis is present at onset, and disability is low (you can walk, you're not disabled already, you only really have one symptom)
- Bad prognosis if...
  - You have rapid progression of many symptoms, can't walk, already have disability

Multiple Sclerosis

- Internuclear Ophthalmoplegia may classically be seen in MS
  - E.g. when looking to the left, the right eye can't adduct across midline, and the left eye shows nystagmus (right-sided internuclear ophthalmoplegia)

- Due to medial longitudinal fasciculus (MLF) lesion
- MLF connects the abducens complex of contralateral side with the CN3 nucleus of ipsilateral side

- **Lhermitte Sign may also classically be seen in MS**
  - Passive neck flexion causes shooting, electric pain in neck and shoulders
  - This is essentially a dural tension test, irritating the already-irritated myelin of these patients

Multiple Sclerosis

- **Diagnosis**
  - Criteria can be heavily detailed (MRI and clinical criteria)
  - Typically we say the patient must have lesions in both space and time
  - This means that we must see more than 1 lesion on MRI in an MS-typical CNS region, and more than 1 clinical attack over time
  - MS CNS regions: spinal cord + 3 brain regions
  - CSF studies may show oligoclonal IgG bands (markers of CNS inflammation)
  - Visual evoked potentials may be abnormal

- **Treatment**
  - High-dose IV corticosteroids for acute attacks +/- plasmapheresis
  - Interferon beta
  - Large amount of immunomodulatory agents that is beyond the scope of a physiatrist

Multiple Sclerosis

- **Rehab considerations**
  - MS patients commonly have central fatigue
  - This means that their "gas tank" starts at a lower level than normal individuals, and will run out earlier in the day than others
  - Submaximal exercise is recommended
  - Sometimes we add neurostimulation to increase their overall dopamine stores and improve energy and alertness
    - Amantadine
    - Methylphenidate
    - Modafinil
  - MS patients are often heat-intolerant, so try to maintain appropriate temperatures for them

Phew! You've done an excellent job getting through a very large chapter (the largest in this book!). It's all downhill from here!

Chapter 5: Musculoskeletal Medicine
Shoulder

The Shoulder

- Ball and socket joint, thus:

- Lots of mobility (flexion and abduction both about 180°)

- ...and plenty of instability (shoulder dislocations)

- You have ligaments and muscles to keep the ball in the socket

- Trauma, excessive eccentric loading (stretching the muscle while it tries to contract), and overuse can damage these ligaments and muscles to cause dislocations and tears

- The 180° of motion happens due to 60° of scapulothoracic motion combined with 120° of glenohumeral motion
  - It's not ALL just the ball moving in the socket to achieve 180°

Shoulder Ligaments

- These are all static stabilizers of the shoulder (they don't move)

- Labrum, shoulder capsule, acromioclavicular (AC) ligament, coracoclavicular (CC) ligament, glenohumeral ligaments

- **Labrum:** rim of fibrocartilage around the glenoid fossa (socket) that functions to deepen the glenoid fossa to improve articulation of the ball within the socket
  - Glenohumeral ligaments, long head of biceps, shoulder capsule attach to the labrum

- **Glenohumeral capsule:** thin, weak, fibrosynovial wrapping around the joint space
  - Serves to actually encapsulate the joint

- **AC ligament:** horizontal ligament connecting acromion to clavicle

- **CC ligament:** ligament connecting coracoid process to clavicle

Shoulder Ligaments

- **Glenohumeral ligaments**

- They are formed from the shoulder capsule tissue, attaching to the glenoid

- This prevents movement/translation of the humeral head on the glenoid
  - They prevent dislocations

- **Superior glenohumeral ligament:** prevents inferior translation

- **Middle glenohumeral ligament:** prevents anterior translation

- **Inferior glenohumeral ligament:** prevents anterior translation above 90°

- If these ligaments are loose, you are "double-jointed", "lax", "hypermobile"
  - May be more prone to MSK pain

Neuromuscular Overview

- Your shoulder abducts, adducts, flexes, extends, internally rotates, and externally rotates
- Lots of muscles perform multiple tasks, but we will cover the main points

Shoulder Abduction

- Supraspinatus: first 15 degrees
  - C5-C6 upper trunk, suprascapular nerve
  - Originates atop the spine of the scapula (SUPRA-SPINE), inserts onto greater tuberosity
- Deltoid: remaining ROM
  - C5-C6 upper trunk, posterior cord, axillary nerve
  - Originates on clavicle, acromion, spine of scapula - inserts onto humerus

Shoulder Adduction

- Pectoralis major
  - C5-T1, all 3 trunks, medial and lateral cords, medial and lateral pectoral nerves
- Latissimus dorsi (lats)
  - C6,C7,C8, all 3 trunks, posterior cord, thoracodorsal nerve
- Teres major
  - Lats and teres major do the same thing: adduct and internally rotate

Shoulder Flexion

- Anterior deltoid
  - C5,C6, upper trunk, posterior cord, axillary nerve
- Biceps brachii
  - C5,C6, upper trunk, lateral cord, musculocutaneous nerve
  - Short head → coracoid process
  - Long head → supraglenoid tuberosity
- Pec major
  - C5-T1 (all roots), all trunks, medial and lateral cord, medial and lateral pectoral nerves

Shoulder Extension

- Triceps
  - Long head mostly (attaches to infraglenoid tuberosity)
  - C6,C7,C8, all 3 trunks, posterior cord, radial nerve
- Rear deltoid

- C5,C6, upper trunk, posterior cord, axillary nerve
- Latissimus dorsi
  - C6,C7,C8, all 3 trunks, posterior cord, thoracodorsal nerve
- Teres major
  - C6,C6, posterior cord, lower subscapular nerve
  - Again, it does whatever the lats do

Shoulder Internal Rotation

- Subscapularis
  - C5,C6, posterior cord, upper and lower subscapular nerves
- Latissimus dorsi
  - C6,C7,C8, all 3 trunks, posterior cord, thoracodorsal nerve
- Teres major
  - C6,C6, posterior cord, lower subscapular nerve
  - Again, it does whatever the lats do

Shoulder External Rotation

- Infraspinatus
  - C5,C6, upper trunk, suprascapular nerve
  - This nerve wraps around the spinoglenoid notch, *then* innervates the infraspinatus
- Teres minor
  - C5,C6, upper trunk, posterior cord, axillary nerve
  - Same innervation as deltoid
- Rear deltoid
  - C5,C6, upper trunk, posterior cord, axillary nerve

Shoulder Joint Arthritis (Glenohumeral Arthritis)

- Osteoarthritis of the shoulder (degenerative joint disease)
- Wear and tear over time, with heavy manual labor, etc.
- This wear and tear grinds down the cartilage, leading to "bone on bone"
- Movement in any plane can cause deep shoulder pain, usually internal rotation and abduction
- Often hurts to palpate the joint

Shoulder Joint Arthritis (Glenohumeral Arthritis)

- **<u>Diagnosis</u>**
  - ○ Physical exam, palpation
  - ○ Xrays
    - ■ Joint space narrowing
    - ■ Osteophytes
    - ■ Cortical irregularities

- **<u>Treatment</u>**
  - ○ Rehab, ibuprofen, acetaminophen, steroid injection into the joint
  - ○ If too painful and the above fails, consider surgery (TSA)
  - ○ Postop: sling, limited ROM leading to Codman PROM exercises and onward

Acromioclavicular Joint Arthritis (AC Joint)

- Connects the acromion of the scapula to the clavicle
- Held together by the **AC ligament**, **CC ligament**, CA ligaments
- Arthritis occurs by wear and tear, overuse, father time
- Scarf test crunches the joint together
- Can use xray and ultrasound to see cortical irregularities, joint space fluid/inflammation, joint space narrowing
- Treatment
  - ○ Rehab, ibuprofen, acetaminophen, ice
  - ○ Corticosteroid injection into the AC joint

AC Joint Separation

- AC joint separation happens when the clavicle separates from the acromion
- Usually due to trauma/FOOSH
- You have to tear the AC ligament to do this
- The CC ligament is 2nd in line to tear
  - ○ If this tears, you have vertical displacement of the clavicle - ouch!
- Types 1-6 (next slide)

AC Joint Separation

- **Type 1**: partial AC tear, intact CC → **rehab**
- **Type 2**: complete AC tear, partial CC tear → **rehab**
- **Type 3**: complete AC tear, complete CC tear → clavicle floats upward and you should **consider surgery**

- **Type 4**: complete AC tear, complete CC tear → clavicle floats up and back, and you need **surgery**
- **Type 5**: complete AC tear, complete CC tear → clavicle floats super up and back, and you need **surgery**
- **Type 6**: complete AC tear, complete CC tear → clavicle floats down, and you need **surgery**

Clavicle Fracture

- Typically due to trauma, most commonly at the **middle third of the clavicle**
- Symptoms: pain, swelling, discoloration over clavicle
- **Diagnosis**: exam, xrays
    - Don't forget to include the joints above and below the injured bone
        - Include SC and AC joints
- **Treatment:** Reduce --> immobilize in sling for 3-6 weeks → ROM → PT
- Surgical referral if open fracture, very displaced clavicle, or significantly abnormal appearance of shoulder

Proximal Humerus Fracture

- Typically due to trauma
- Symptoms: arm pain, swelling, shoulder disfigurement, weakness, sensory disturbance
- **Diagnosis:** xrays
- Four-part fracture classification system
    - One-part: humerus is still in one part, i.e. nondisplaced impaction
    - Two-part: one part is displaced from the remainder of the humerus
    - Three-part: two fragments are displaced from the humerus (the third "part")
    - Four-part: four fragments exist
- These parts are the greater tuberosity, lesser tuberosity, humeral head, humeral shaft
- Most fractures occur at the surgical neck, hence the name

Proximal Humerus Fracture

- **Treatment**
    - One-part fracture: sling x6 weeks → PT (Codman, pendulum exercises)
    - 2-4 part fracture: surgery (ORIF)
- Check radial pulse
- Check neuro exam
- **Axillary nerve may be injured** in surgical neck fracture

- Impaired deltoid, teres minor (abduction, external rotation), sensation over lateral shoulder/arm
- Radial nerve typically is injured in midshaft humeral fractures, so should be spared here

Humeral Stress Fracture

- Typically occurs due to repetitive overuse, e.g. pitchers, throwers
- Humeral growth plate may become damaged in kids; otherwise stress fractures form at the humeral shaft
- Symptoms: shoulder pain worse with throwing
- Diagnosis: tender to palpation over fracture site, pain with resisted shoulder movements, xrays/MRI
- Treatment: shut it down! Limit activity for 8-12 weeks
  - May gradually increase throwing activity after it has healed (symptoms, xrays)

Shoulder Dislocations

- The shoulder has lots of ROM, thus making it unstable
- We use different terms to describe how much instability is really taking place:
  - **Instability:** the humeral head moves around (translates) in the glenoid fossa
  - **Subluxation:** the humeral head actually pops out of the glenoid but then immediately returns
  - **Dislocation:** the humeral head pops out and stays there
- Typically dislocations happen in the anterior direction (**anterior inferior**)
- Happens in the position of abduction and external rotation
  - Like winding up to throw a baseball
  - Same position as our anterior apprehension test
  - Tends to recur
- Posterior dislocations happen rarely, in a flexed, adducted arm (opposite of anterior dislocation position)
  - This flexed, adducted position is also the same position we use for our posterior instability testing

TUBS and AMBRI

- Sound like government spy agencies, but alas...
- They are simply useful mnemonics to remember how to manage dislocations
- **TUBS**
  - Traumatic
  - Unidirectional, Unilateral
  - Bankart lesions coexist

- o   Surgery
- **AMBRI**
  - o   Atraumatic
  - o   Multidirectional (i.e. these patients are generally very flexible = = ligamentous laxity)
  - o   Bilateral
  - o   Rehab
  - o   Inferior capsular shift if they require surgery

Bankart and Hill-Sachs Lesions

- Both are associated with anterior dislocations
- **Bankart lesion:** anterior labral tear
  - o   Thus, labrum is torn, so dislocation is likely to happen in that anterior direction we talked about
- **Hill-Sachs lesion:** Posterolateral humeral head compression fracture
  - o   If the humeral head is compressed and its articulation with the glenoid is no longer good, then you will have instability
  - o   You can see a notch on the posterolateral humeral head on xrays

Physical Exam for Instability

- **Anterior apprehension test**
  - o   Lie patient flat on their back, then abduct and externally rotate their arm
  - o   Finally, put your hand under their midhumeral shaft area and push it upward toward the ceiling
  - o   If test is positive, the patient will have pain or sudden fear that their shoulder is dislocating (apprehension!)
- **Jerk and Kim tests** for posterior instability
  - o   **Jerk:** flex arm to 90 and internally rotate, then adduct arm across body while pushing humerus posteriorly (i.e. trying to dislocate the humerus posteriorly to see if they are truly susceptible to this). The patient will **jerk** away if possible.
  - o   **Kim:** similar, but flex arm upward and apply a posteroinferiorly directed force. Don't have to adduct the arm across the body or internally rotate for this.

Diagnosis and Treatment of Instability

- Physical exam: anterior apprehension, Jerk, Kim
- Xrays
- MR arthrogram is useful if you want to prove a labral tear exists
  - o   Dye will flow into the labral defect and show up white on the images
- Treatment: TUBS and AMBRI

- In general, have to fail rehab in order to get surgery

Labral Tear

- **Labrum:** cartilage that extends out and circles around the glenoid fossa, thus deepening the socket so the humerus can better articulate with the glenoid

- Injured by repetitive overhead activity or trauma

- **Diagnosis:** O'Brien test, xrays, MR arthrogram
    - **O'Brien** test: hold arm out, palm down, adducted a little bit towards midline. Then push down on patient's arm while they try to resist.
    - A positive test is more painful with palm down resistance than with palm up

Adhesive Capsulitis (Frozen Shoulder)

- Shoulder capsule becomes extremely restricting and tight

- Happens usually after trauma, stroke, or some type of inflammation

- Patient cannot range their shoulder well (very tight and painful)
    - Abduction and external rotation are restricted first
    - Usually painful for several months, then incredibly stiff for several months, then these both gradually improve

- **Diagnosis:** history and physical exam (ROM), xrays, MR arthrogram

- **Treatment:** PT, steroid injections into GHJ and subAC bursa space
    - Suprascapular nerve block followed by high-volume injection of lidocaine, steroid, saline combination into GHJ under US guidance. Can be very effective.
    - Take to OR and try to manually break up the contracture
    - Arthroscopic surgery

Rotator Cuff Tear

- **Rotator cuff** = 4 muscles that are the true reason why the ball stays in the socket

- Supraspinatus: initial abduction

- Infraspinatus: external rotation

- Teres minor: external rotation

- Subscapularis: internal rotation

- Usually you tear the supraspinatus
    - Pain with overhead activities, especially >60 degrees abduction
    - Sleeping on that arm hurts

- If it's not completely torn, rehab it

- If it's completely torn, have surgical repair

- If rehab is too painful, try corticosteroid + lidocaine injection
- Consider regenerative medicine, e.g. PRP

Rotator Cuff Tear

- **Diagnosis**
  - Empty can
  - Full can
  - Drop arm test
  - Neer
  - Hawkins
  - Test external rotation, belly lift-off as well for the other muscles
  - Xray: can see changes in the tendon as it inserts onto the humerus
  - MRI: much better for soft tissue (i.e. muscle) diagnosis than xray
  - Ultrasound: quick, in-office, dynamic visualization of soft and bony tissues
    - Can also target specific structures at that moment if you wish (e.g. bursae)
    - Check biceps tendon while you're at it; they tend to tear together
    - Can diagnose and treat calcific tendonitis: saline lavage

Scapular Dyskinesis

- Abnormal motion of the scapula, causing back and shoulder pain
- Results from periscapular muscle weakness
  - Serratus anterior, trapezius, rhomboid, levator scapula, pec minor
- Medial and lateral scapular winging
  - **Medial:** serratus anterior is weak, often due to long thoracic nerve injury
  - **Lateral:** trapezius is weak, often due to spinal accessory nerve injury
- Diagnosis: examine scapular mobility
- Treatment: scapular PT
- Note: patient may have rotator cuff pathology due to scapular dyskinesis

Biceps Tendonopathy

- **Tendonopathy:** nonspecific pathology of a tendon
- **Tendonitis:** acute inflammation of a tendon due to microtears
- **Tendonosis:** chronic degeneration due to overuse
- **Biceps tendonopathy:** typically occurs at proximal long head tendon
  - Long head: inserts onto supraglenoid tuberosity
  - Short head inserts onto coracoid process

- Due to repetitive biceps loading, shoulder overuse
- Symptoms: anterior shoulder pain
- **Diagnosis:** Speed/Yergason/Hook/Ludington, MRI, US
- **Treatment:** PT, heat/ice, USG tendon sheath injection, biceps tenodesis
  - With steroid injection, beware biceps tendon rupture

Way to go! You are building the foundation for a really strong grasp of musculoskeletal pathology, starting here with the shoulder. Keep at it and you will be able to answer questions in your sleep.

Chapter 6: Musculoskeletal Medicine
Elbow

The Elbow

- Hinge joint (flexion and extension)

- Not just "humerus and forearm"

  - Radiocapitellar joint (humeroradial joint)

  - Ulnotrochlear joint (humeroulnar joint)

  - Proximal radioulnar joint

- Forearm also able to pronate and supinate

- Bony anatomy and ligaments hold the elbow together

- Trochlea, capitellum, olecranon, olecranon fossa, coronoid process and fossa, RCL, UCL, annular ligament of radius)

- When elbow is extended, it normally has about 5-15° of natural valgus attitude

  - Allows your elbow to clear your body when the elbow is extended

Neuromuscular Overview

- Your elbow flexes, extends, pronates, supinates

- We will cover the main movers

Elbow Flexion

- Biceps brachii

  - C5-C6, upper trunk, lateral cord, musculocutaneous nerve

- **Brachialis**

  - C5-C6, upper trunk, lateral cord, musculocutaneous nerve

- Brachioradialis

  - C5-C6, upper trunk, posterior cord, radial nerve (BELOW the spiral groove)

- Pronator teres

  - C6-C7, upper and middle trunks, lateral cord, median nerve

Elbow Extension

- Triceps

  - C6-C7-C8, all 3 trunks, posterior cord, radial nerve (innervated ABOVE the spiral groove)

- Anconeus

  - C6-C7-C8, all 3 trunks, posterior cord, radial nerve (innervated ABOVE the spiral groove)

Forearm Supination

- **Biceps brachii**
  - C5-C6, upper trunk, lateral cord, musculocutaneous nerve
- Supinator
  - C5-C6, upper trunk, posterior cord, radial nerve, PIN

Forearm Pronation

- Pronator teres
  - C6-C7, upper and middle trunks, lateral cord, median nerve
- Pronator quadratus
  - C7-C8-T1, middle and lower trunks, medial and lateral cords, median nerve, AIN

Common Flexor Tendon

- Located at medial epicondyle of humerus (golfer's elbow / medial epicondylitis)
- Pronator teres (PT)
  - C6-C7, upper and middle trunks, lateral cord, median nerve
- Flexor carpi radialis (FCR)
  - C6-C7, upper and middle trunks, lateral cord, median nerve
- Palmaris longus
- Flexor carpi ulnaris (FCU)
  - C8-T1, lower trunk, medial cord, ulnar nerve
- Flexor digitorum superficialis (FDS)
  - C7-C8, middle and lower trunks, medial and lateral cords, median nerve
- Flexor digitorum profundus (FDP)
  - C7-C8-T1, middle and lower trunks, medial cord, AIN / ulnar nerve
  - So "profound" that it requires 2 nerves to innervate it (median and ulnar)

Common Extensor Tendon

- Located at lateral epicondyle of humerus
  - Inflammation causes tennis elbow (lateral epicondylitis)
- Extensor carpi radialis longus and brevis (ECRL, **ECRB**)
- Extensor digitorum (ED/EDC)
  - C7-C8, middle and lower trunk, posterior cord, radial nerve, PIN
- Anconeus
  - C6-C7-C8, all 3 trunks, posterior cord, radial nerve (ABOVE the spiral groove)

- Supinator
- Extensor carpi ulnaris (ECU)
  - C7-C8, middle and lower trunk, posterior cord, radial nerve, PIN

Humeral Shaft Fracture

- Usually due to trauma, FOOSH
- Painful, swollen arm
- Workup: xrays, physical exam (good neurovascular exam)
- Treatment: splinting in vast majority of cases
- Remember: **radial nerve injury**!

Distal Humerus Fracture

- Usually due to trauma
- Painful, swollen elbow
- Workup: xrays, physical exam (good neurovascular exam)
- Treatment: splinting (nondisplaced) vs. ORIF (displaced)

Olecranon Fracture

- Usually due to trauma, FOOSH
- Painful, swollen elbow
- Workup: xrays, physical exam
- Treatment: splinting (nondisplaced) vs. ORIF (displaced)
- Beware **ulnar nerve injury**!

Radial Head Fracture

- Usually due to trauma, FOOSH
- Painful, swollen elbow
- Workup: xrays, physical exam (decreased elbow ROM)
- Treatment: splinting (nondisplaced), ORIF (displaced or comminuted)

Valgus Extension Overload Syndrome (VEO)

- Caused by excessive, repetitive valgus extension forces
  - Baseball pitchers
- Posteromedial elbow pain worse with pitching and the VEO test
  - **VEO test:** flex elbow, then extend it while applying a valgus stress (this simulates the pitching motion under stress)

- Workup: xrays (olecranon osteophytes or loose bodies can be seen)
- Treatment: Surgery to remove the above. Fix pitching mechanics.
- **Little Leaguer's Elbow:** repetitive valgus stress in pitcher, leading to traction apophysitis of the medial epicondyle, leading to osteochondritis dissecans of the capitellum

Osteochondrosis of the Elbow

- Aseptic necrosis of the capitellum epiphysis due to poor blood supply to the epiphysis
- Lateral elbow pain worse with activity, improved with rest
  - Happens usually in children
- Workup: xrays (patchy lucencies in the capitellum)
- Treatment: splinting, then gradually increase activity

Elbow Dislocation

- Usually due to trauma, FOOSH
- Most common dislocation in children
  - Shoulder in adults
- Posterior dislocation is the usual direction
- Workup: xrays, physical exam (good neurovascular exam)
- Treatment: closed reduction → splinting → gradually increase activity

Nursemaid Elbow

- Radial head subluxes out of place due to being yanked out of the annular ligament's grasp
- Usually due to someone yanking upward on a child's arm by the hand
- Painful arm, child does not move the arm
- Workup: physical exam, xrays
- Treatment: reduce it: hyperpronate the arm or supinate while flexing the elbow

Ulnar Collateral Ligament Sprain

- AKA medial collateral ligament sprain
- Excessive valgus force causes tearing (sprain) of the anterior bundle of the UCL
- Medial elbow pain with laxity on valgus stress testing
- Workup: physical exam, xrays (calcification or cortical irregularities/spurs along the UCL), ultrasound valgus stress test to demonstrate increased laxity
- Treatment: RICE, PT, surgery (Tommy John)

Radial Collateral Ligament Sprain

- AKA lateral collateral ligament sprain

- Excessive varus force causes tearing (sprain) of RCL

- Pain at lateral elbow, worse with varus stress testing

- Workup: physical exam, xrays, ultrasound to demonstrate joint space widening under varus stress

- Treatment: RICE, PT, surgery

Olecranon Bursitis

- Inflammation of the olecranon bursa at the posterior elbow (olecranon)

- Due to repetitive force to that area (e.g. resting head on elbow)
  - Gout, pseudogout, RA can also be associated with this

- A huge pouch develops at the olecranon because there is little tissue there to restrict it from expanding

- Workup: physical exam, consider aspiration and culture if you suspect infection

- Treatment: RICE, elbow pad, aspiration

Lateral Epicondylitis (Tennis Elbow)

- Common extensor tendonitis/microtearing due to repetitive overuse of the wrist/finger extensors **(usually ECRB)**

- Commonly seen in tennis players

- Pain at common extensor tendon origin at lateral epicondyle
  - **Cozen test:** pain while palpating proximal common extensor tendon with resisted wrist extension
  - **Mill's test:** pain while extending elbow, flexing and radially deviating the wrist (stretching out the common extensor tendon in order to irritate it)

- Workup: physical exam

- Treatment: RICE, PT, splinting, steroid injection, tenotomy, regenerative therapies

- Tennis players: need to increase grip size, decrease string tension to below 55lbs, play on a slow court (e.g. clay), correct technique

Medial Epicondylitis (Golfer Elbow)

- Common flexor tendon inflammation due to repetitive overuse, valgus stresses, resulting in microtearing of common flexor tendon

- Commonly seen in golfers, pitchers

- Pain at common flexor tendon origin at medial epicondyle, worse with resisted wrist flexion, or extension while palpating the common flexor tendon origin

- Workup: physical exam
- Treatment: RICE, splinting, PT, correct throwing/swing mechanics

Distal Biceps Tendonitis/Tear

- Repetitive overload/overuse of the biceps causes inflammation/microtears of the distal biceps tendon as it inserts onto the radial tuberosity
- Pain over antecubital fossa, worse with loading the biceps tendon (e.g. curls)
- If rupture occurs, it is sudden, with sudden onset of swelling and bruising in anterior elbow (obtain xrays in this case to rule out avulsion of bone)
- Hook test: place finger around distal biceps tendon in the anterior elbow, and try to "hook" it out of the elbow. If it's torn, it will give way easily.
- Treatment: RICE, PT, correct technique, surgery if rupture or avulsion

Triceps Tendonitis/Tear

- Pain in posterior elbow/triceps tendon region due to excessive overuse (e.g. repetitive elbow extension), worse with resisted elbow extension
- Avulsion can occur if sudden eccentric force is applied to triceps
- Workup: xrays, physical exam
- Treatment: RICE, PT, surgery if avulsion

Knowing the MSK anatomy and pathology of both shoulder and elbow? If only you could know the wrist and hand as well! Wait a minute...

Chapter 7: Musculoskeletal Medicine
Wrist/Hand

The Wrist

- Very mobile, like the hip and shoulder
  - Uses many bones and muscles to achieve this, rather than ball and socket strategy

- Flexion, extension, ulnar deviation, radial deviation

- Distal radioulnar joint connected together by radioulnar ligaments

- Carpal bones:
DISTAL:	Trapezium	Trapezoid	Capitate	Hamate
PROXIMAL:	Scaphoid	Lunate	Triquetrum	Pisiform

- Ligaments connect carpal bone to carpal bone

Neuromuscular Overview

- As discussed, your wrist performs:

- Flexion, extension, ulnar deviation, radial deviation

- We'll cover the main muscles for each function

Wrist Flexion

- Flexor carpi radialis (FCR)
  - C6-C7, upper and middle trunk, lateral cord, median nerve

- Flexor carpi ulnaris (FCU)
  - C8-T1, lower trunk, medial cord, ulnar nerve

- Flexor digitorum superficialis (FDS) and flexor digitorum profundus (FDP), flexor pollicis longus (FPL), and palmaris longus also provide wrist flexion action to a lesser degree

Wrist Extension

- Extensor carpi radialis longus and brevis (ECRL, ECRB)
  - C6-C7, upper and middle trunk, posterior cord, radial nerve

- Extensor carpi ulnaris (ECU)
  - C7-C8, middle and lower trunk, posterior cord, radial nerve, PIN

- Extensor digitorum (ED), extensor indicis proprius (EIP), extensor pollicis longus (EPL), extensor digiti minimi (EDM) also contribute to a lesser degree

Ulnar Deviation

- FCU
  - C8-T1, lower trunk, medial cord, ulnar nerve

- ECU
  - C7-C8, middle and lower trunk, posterior cord, radial nerve, PIN
- The two ulnar-sided wrist-action muscles

Radial Deviation

- FCR
  - C6-C7, upper and middle trunk, lateral cord, median nerve
- ECRL, ECRB
  - C6-C7, upper and middle trunk, posterior cord, radial nerve

Volar Side of the Wrist (Carpal Tunnel)

- Common site of entrapment of the median nerve
- Carpal tunnel has 10 structures within it:
  - 4 FDS tendons, 4 FDP tendons, FPL tendon, median nerve
- All under the flexor retinaculum
- Carpal tunnel inlet is bordered by the scaphoid and pisiform (radially and ulnarly)

Dorsal Side of the Wrist

- Wrist and finger extensors pass through 6 compartments, going radial to ulnar
- 1st: APL, EPB
- 2nd: ECRL, ECRB
- 3rd: EPL
- 4th: ED, EIP
- 5th: EDM
- 6th: ECU
- Repetition!

Osteoarthritis of the Wrist

- "Wear and tear" of articular cartilage in the wrist
  - Causes bone to grind against bone
  - Sclerosis of bone surfaces as this occurs
  - Osteophytes
- Heberden nodes: DIP appears swollen due to osteophytes
- 1st CMC arthritis is very common
  - 1st CMC grind test: grind the thumb around like a mortar and pestle to reproduce their thumb pain

Distal Radius Fracture

- Due to trauma, FOOSH

- Painful, swollen wrist

- Fracture happens in two different ways:

- **Colles Fracture:** distal radius fragment is dorsally displaced (**CD**)

- **Smith Fracture:** distal radius fragment is volarly displaced (**S**weater **V**est)

- Workup: physical exam, xrays

- Treatment: ortho referral

Scaphoid Fracture

- Usually due to trauma, FOOSH

- Pain in anatomic snuffbox is classic
  - Snuffbox borders: scaphoid (base/floor), APL/EPB (lateral), EPL (medial)

- Workup: physical exam, xrays, CT/MRI

- Treatment: immobilize with thumb spica cast, repeat xrays in 2 weeks if initial xrays were negative but you still suspect scaphoid fracture, consider surgery if proximal ⅓ fracture or if fracture is displaced

- **Most common at scaphoid waist**

- **Proximal ⅓ of scaphoid has highest risk of AVN**

Kienbock Disease / Osteonecrosis of the Lunate

- Idiopathic AVN of the lunate (the bone dies due to poor blood supply)

- Pain over the dorsal wrist (ulnar to the snuffbox)

- Workup: physical exam, xrays, MRI

- Treatment: surgery

Hamate Fracture

- Usually due to trauma, FOOSH

- Site of pain (hamate) is distal to the ulnar-sided bump (pisiform) on your own volar wrist

- Pain over the hamate, worse with swinging a bat or golf club, or applying axial pressure to the 4th/5th digits

- Workup: physical exam, xrays, CT

- Treatment: immobilize in short arm cast (nondisplaced), surgery (displaced)

Ganglion Cyst

- Small pouch of synovial fluid that comes out of the joint space or tendon sheath
  - Basically a synovial herniation out of the joint
- Usually found on the dorsum of the wrist
- Workup: physical exam, ultrasound, xrays (normal), MRI
- Treatment: observation, aspiration, surgery

De Quervain Tenosynovitis

- 1st compartment synovitis due to repetitive overuse of the APL, EPB
- Pain over the 1st compartment
- Finkelstein test: place thumb in palm, then ulnar deviate the wrist
  - Positive if this reproduces their pain
  - Usually very painful!
- Workup: physical exam
- Treatment: NSAIDs, thumb spica splint for immobilization, tendon sheath injection (with/without US guidance), surgery for tendon sheath release

The Hand

- The hand is made up of (surprise) bones, ligaments, tendons, nerves, and blood vessels
- The bones are the 5 metacarpals, 5 proximal phalanges, 4 middle phalanges (the thumb does not have one), and 5 distal phalanges
- Major ligaments are the MCLs and LCLs of all of these joints
- The tendons are the flexor digitorum superficialis and profundus tendons on the flexor side of the hand, and extensor tendons on the dorsal side of the hand
- The hand is mostly ulnar-innervated, except for the 1/2 LOAF muscles (median)
- The blood supply to the hand is via the radial and ulnar arteries
- The thumb and fingers abduct (dorsal interossei), adduct (palmar interossei), flex (FDS/FDP/FPL/etc.), and extend (ED/EIP/EPL/etc.)

Finger Abduction and Adduction

- Finger abduction is performed by the dorsal interossei (DAB)
  - Innervated by the ulnar nerve
- Finger adduction is performed by the palmar interossei (PAD)
  - Innervated by the ulnar nerve
- We have 3 PADs and 4 DABs

Finger Flexion

- Finger flexion is performed at the PIPs and DIPs

- PIP flexion is performed by the flexor digitorum superficialis (FDS)
    - C7-C8, middle and lower trunk, medial and lateral cord, median nerve

- DIP flexion is performed by the flexor digitorum profundus (FDP)
    - C7-C8-T1, middle and lower trunk, medial cord, median nerve, AIN
        - For FDP to digits 2 and 3
    - C7-C8-T1, middle and lower trunk, medial cord, ulnar nerve
        - For FDP to digits 4 and 5

- Thumb flexion is performed by the flexor pollicis brevis (FPB) and flexor pollicis longus (FPL)
    - FPL: C7-C8-T1, middle and lower trunk, medial and lateral cord, median nerve, AIN
    - FPB: C8-T1, lower trunk, medial cord, median AND ulnar nerve

Finger Extension

- Finger extension is performed by the extensor digitorum (ED), extensor indicis proprius (EIP), extensor pollicis longus (EPL), and extensor digiti minimi (EDM)

- Digit 2-5 extension is performed by the ED
    - The ED actually attaches to a thick piece of tissue called the extensor expansion which pulls on both the DIPs and PIPs, causing extension of both
    - Thus, you don't have an "extensor digitorum superficialis" and "profundus" - just the one ED
    - C7-C8, middle and lower trunk, posterior cord, radial nerve, PIN

- Digit 2 (index finger) extension is achieved the same way by the EIP
    - C7-C8, middle and lower trunk, posterior cord, radial nerve, PIN

- Thumb extension is performed by the EPL

- Digit 5 extension (the pinky) is performed by the EDM

Thumb Motion

- The thumb can perform flexion, extension, palmar abduction, radial abduction, opposition, apposition, adduction

Metacarpal Neck/Shaft Fracture

- "Boxer's Fracture" - occurs after punching something hard, usually 5th metacarpal

- Pain over fractured metacarpal

- Workup: physical exam, xrays

- Treatment: ortho referral (management can be conservative or surgical)

Skier's Thumb / 1st UCL Injury

- Injury of the ulnar collateral ligament (UCL) of the MCP of the thumb due to excessive radial deviation which tears the ligament

- Workup: physical exam (laxity and pain in palmar abduction), xrays

- Treatment: immobilize thumb in spica splint to allow ligament to heal

- Note: Stener's lesion is trapping of the thumb adductor aponeurosis in the MCP joint due to a severe UCL tear that opens up access to the joint. This needs ortho referral for possible surgery

MCP/PIP/DIP Collateral Ligament Injury

- Usually due to excessive varus or valgus deviation due to sports (basketball, tennis, baseball)

- Painful, swollen joint

- Workup: physical exam (varus/valgus stress testing), xrays to rule out fracture/dislocation

- Treatment: buddy tape the finger or apply extension splint to the finger

Dupuytren Contracture

- Palmar fascia thickens into fibrous cords

- Leads to painless swelling and flexion contracture of usually the ring finger

- Usually older men with seizures/diabetes/alcoholism

- Workup: physical exam

- Treatment: OT, steroid injection, surgery

Trigger Finger

- Stenosing tenosynovitis at the A1 (MCP) pulley of a finger flexor

- Nodule forms at the A1 pulley, preventing flexor tendon from gliding through smoothly

- Finger tends to snap and catch when flexing/extending

- Workup: physical exam

- Treatment: observation, splinting, NSAIDs, steroid injection into tendon sheath, surgery

Jersey Finger

- FDS or FDP tendon avulsion due to sudden hyperextension of the digit, e.g. getting caught in a player's jersey

- Pain and swelling in finger/palm; inability to flex the PIP or DIP

- Workup: physical exam (test FDS and FDP separately), xrays to rule out avulsion of bone with the tendon

- Treatment: ortho referral for surgery

Mallet Finger

- Sudden DIP flexion can cause extensor tendon rupture, possibly with bony fragment coming off with it (avulsion fracture)

- Painful, swollen distal finger with inability to extend DIP

- Workup: physical exam, xrays

- Treatment: DIP extension splint to allow tendon to heal for several weeks, followed by ROM; surgery if big avulsed bone fragment

Woohoo! That does it for MSK of the upper extremity! Think of what could possibly come next... Maybe even the lower extremity! The anticipation!

Chapter 8: Musculoskeletal Medicine
Hip/Pelvis

Don't Forget

- The pelvis, hips, knees, ankles, and feet are all connected by the same kinetic chain starting in the feet

- Dysfunction of one part can lead to dysfunction and pain in other parts

- Consider that rehabbing knee pain also must consist of core and hip girdle strengthening. A stable pelvis means stable control of the knee.

The Pelvis

- Consists of the ileum, ischium, pubis, and sacrum

- Important joints include the sacroiliac joint (SI joint) and pubic symphysis

- We will cover SI joint pathology in the spine section

The Hip

- Very mobile ball and socket joint consisting of the femur and acetabulum (femoroacetabular joint)

- Flexion, extension, abduction, adduction, internal rotation, external rotation

- Lots of ROM means higher risk for dislocation

- Bony articulation, ligaments, and muscles keep everything in place

Hip Bony Anatomy

- Ball and socket (femur and acetabulum)

- Articular cartilage for smooth gliding and cushioning

- If abnormal, may lead to hip impingement (femoroacetabular impingement)

Hip Ligaments

- Iliofemoral ligament
    - Extends from ileum to femur on anterior part of hip
    - **Strongest ligament in the body**
    - **Limits abduction, extension, external rotation**

- Pubofemoral ligament
    - Extends from pubis to femur on anterior part of hip
    - Limits abduction

- Ischiofemoral ligament
    - Extends from ischium to femur on posterior part of hip

- o   Limits internal rotation

Hip Ligaments

- Hip joint capsule
  - o   Extends from acetabulum down to intertrochanteric crest to encapsulate the ball and socket
- Labrum
  - o   Lip of cartilage that rings around the acetabular ridge to deepen the ball within the socket
- Ligamentum capitis femoris
  - o   Ligament of the head of the femur
  - o   Extends from acetabulum into the femoral head and carries blood supply to that area

Neuromuscular Overview

- Your hip performs flexion, extension, abduction, adduction, internal rotation, external rotation
- Let's cover the major nerves and muscles that allow this to happen

Hip Flexion

- Iliopsoas
  - o   L2, L3, L4, femoral nerve
- Sartorius
  - o   L2, L3, L4, femoral nerve
- Rectus femoris
  - o   L2, L3, L4, femoral nerve

Hip Extension

- Gluteus maximus
  - o   L5, S1, S2, inferior gluteal nerve
- Gluteus medius (posterior fibers)
  - o   L4, L5, S1, superior gluteal nerve
- Semimembranosus, semitendinosus
  - o   L4, L5, S1, sciatic nerve (tibial division)
- Biceps femoris
  - o   L5, S1, sciatic nerve (tibial division for long head / fibular division for short head)

Hip Abduction

- Gluteus medius
  - L4, L5, S1, superior gluteal nerve
- Gluteus minimus
  - L4, L5, S1, superior gluteal nerve
- Tensor fascia lata (TFL)
  - L4, L5, S1, superior gluteal nerve

Hip Adduction

- Adductor longus, magnus, brevis
  - L2, L3, L4, obturator nerve (magnus has some sciatic nerve [tibial division] innervation)
- Gracilis
  - L2, L3, L4, obturator nerve
- Pectineus
  - L2, L3, L4, femoral nerve

Hip Internal Rotation

- Adductor longus, magnus, brevis
  - L2, L3, L4, obturator nerve (magnus has some sciatic nerve [tibial division] innervation)
- Tensor fascia lata (TFL)
  - L4, L5, S1, superior gluteal nerve
- Gluteus medius and minimus
  - L4, L5, S1, superior gluteal nerve
- Semimembranosus, semitendinosus
  - L4, L5, S1, sciatic nerve (tibial division)

Hip External Rotation

- Piriformis
- Superior gemellus ("GOGO" muscles)
- Obturator internus
- Inferior gemellus
- Obturator externus
- Quadratus femoris
- Gluteus maximus

      o   L5, S1, S2, inferior gluteal nerve

Hip Osteoarthritis

- Degeneration of articular cartilage due to wear and tear (not inflammation!)
- Reactive sclerosis, subchondral cysts, decreased joint space all develop
- Internal rotation is lost first with superolateral compartment narrowing
- Pain in the **groin** reflects true hip joint pain
- FABERE, FAIR, hip scour, log roll will elicit ipsilateral groin pain
- **Workup:** xrays
- **Treatment:** cane, walker, shoe orthotics, PT, corticosteroid injection, THA

Leg Length Discrepancy

- Patients present with back and hip/groin pain, functional scoliosis
- **True** leg length discrepancy
  - Measure distance from ASIS to medial malleolus on both sides, and compare
  - CT scanogram is most accurate test
- **Apparent** leg length discrepancy
  - Due to oblique position of pelvis or inappropriate leg position
  - Measure distance from umbilicus to medial malleolus on both sides
- **Treatment:** observation, shoe lifts, surgery

Hip Dislocation

- Typically happens in the posterior direction, in a dashboard MVA injury
  - Exactly the position you want to avoid if you are post-op from posterior approach hip replacement surgery (flexion past 90 degrees, adduction past midline, internal rotation)
    - This position puts the hip particularly at risk for a posterior dislocation
- If posterior dislocation, consider sciatic nerve injury
- If anterior dislocation, consider femoral nerve injury
- Pain in groin with shorter-appearing leg
- **Workup:** xrays (dislocated hip appears higher than the other)
- **Treatment:** stat ortho consult (AVN and major nerves are at risk) for either closed reduction or operative intervention

Femoral Neck Fracture (Intracapsular)

- Usually due to fall in elderly patient
- More likely if: osteoporosis, female, elderly, white, taking steroids, smoking, low BMI, poor nutrition
- Occurs within the hip capsule (extends from acetabulum down to femoral neck)
- Garden Classification System
  - Stage 1: incomplete fracture line, nondisplaced
  - Stage 2: complete fracture line (all the way across the bone), nondisplaced
  - Stage 3: complete and partially displaced
  - Stage 4: complete and fully displaced (capsule completely torn)
- **Workup:** xrays (applying Garden Classification above)
- **Treatment:** usually ORIF
- Hip precautions post-op; avoid extremes of motion

Intertrochanteric Hip Fracture

- Most common hip fracture
- Extracapsular
- Occurs in the region just distal to femoral neck, between the two trochanters
- Pain in groin with an externally rotated, shortened leg
- **Workup:** xrays, CT/MRI
- **Treatment:** ORIF

Subtrochanteric Hip Fracture

- Fracture in the proximal femur below the intertrochanteric region
- Pain in groin with limb shortened and externally rotated
- **Workup:** xrays
- **Treatment:** ORIF

Proximal Femoral Stress Fracture

- Stress reaction of bone, leading to a split/fracture of the bone that shows up as a line of lucency on xrays
- Groin pain due to doing too much, too far, too fast (overtraining)
  - At risk if low BMI, poor nutrition, amenorrhea, osteoporosis (female athlete triad)
- **Workup:** xrays, bone scan (if xrays negative)
- **Compression-side fracture**

- ○ More common and stable
- ○ Located along inferior femoral neck
- ○ Can be rehabbed (NWB → WBAT → gradually increase activity)
- ○ ORIF
- **Tension-side fracture**
  - ○ Less stable
  - ○ Located along superior femoral neck
  - ○ Requires ORIF

Slipped Capital Femoral Epiphysis (SCFE)

- Slipping of the metaphysis under the epiphysis
- Classically occurs in obese adolescent males
- Groin pain worse with walking
  - ○ Trendelenburg (antalgic) gait
- **Workup:** xrays
  - ○ Grade 1: <33% slippage
  - ○ Grade 2: 33-50% slippage
  - ○ Grade 3: >50% slippage
- **Treatment:** ORIF
- Consider endocrine referral for GH deficiency, thyroid disease

Femoroacetabular Impingement (FAI)

- Abnormal contact between the femur and acetabulum during ROM
- Causes groin pain with activity, usually in young, athletic males
- Due to CAM and/or Pincer lesions
- **CAM lesion**
  - ○ Essentially a larger head/neck region of the femur
  - ○ Essentially a "knuckle" of bone coming out of the femoral neck
- **Pincer lesion**
  - ○ Acetabulum extends too far, and "pincers" the femoral head/neck on ROM
- Labral tears often occur due to this
- **Workup:** xrays, MRI, MR arthrogram
- **Treatment:** PT, corticosteroid/regenerative injection, surgery

Avascular Necrosis of the Femoral Head (AVN)

- Gradual onset of pain in groin, secondary to poor, severely decreased blood supply to the femoral head due to a variety of issues
    - Congenital (Legg-Calve-Perthes disease)
    - Excessive corticosteroid usage
    - Alcohol
    - SLE (lupus)
- **Workup:** xrays, MRI (dark area on T1; bright on T2)
- **Treatment:** surgery

Osteitis Pubis

- Pubic symphysis inflammation due to repetitive adductor overuse
- Vague pain in the groin, very proximal medial thigh (adductor origin)
- Pain with resisted adduction or palpating proximal adductors while abducting the thigh; pain with direct pubic symphysis palpation
- **Workup:** xrays (osteolytic pubic bone with erosions of the bone, sometimes diastasis of the joint), MRI, bone scan shows increased uptake at pubic symphysis bones
- **Treatment:** rest, ice, NSAIDs, PT, corticosteroid injection

Hip Labral Tear

- Disruption of the rim of cartilage surrounding the acetabulum
- Usually due to trauma, FAI
- Vague groin pain, worse with ROM, associated with clicking/snapping/locking, often worse at extremes of ROM (e.g. extreme hip flexion)
- **Workup:** xrays (look for bony displasia), MR arthrogram (will see white dye flowing into the labral tear - labrum will appear uniformly dark in normal patient)
- **Treatment:** PT, injection (PRP), surgery

Ischial Bursitis

- Pain over ischia ("sit bones") with sitting, due to inflammation of the ischial bursa, which lies between the ischial tuberosity and the gluteus maximus muscle
- The ischial tuberosity is also the origin of the hamstrings
- Can be due to overuse, inflammation, trauma
- **Workup:** xrays, MRI, US
- **Treatment:** rest, ice, NSAIDs, PT, US-guided corticosteroid injection

Iliopsoas Bursitis and Tendonitis

- Groin pain due to inflammation of the iliopsoas tendon or bursa due to repetitive overuse of the iliopsoas (hip flexion)
- Associated with internal snapping hip syndrome
- **Workup:** none or xrays, US
- **Treatment:** rest, ice, NSAIDs, PT, US-guided corticosteroid/PRP injection

Internal Snapping Hip

- Groin pain caused by the iliopsoas tendon subluxing/snapping over the iliopectineal eminence
- Can be associated with iliopsoas bursitis/tendonitis
- Pain, snapping, clicking in the groin with extension, abduction, external rotation
- If patient complains of snapping sensation in groin, they probably have this
- **Workup:** none, xray, US
- **Treatment:** rest, ice, NSAIDs, PT, US-guided corticosteroid/PRP

External Snapping Hip

- Pain in lateral thigh over the greater trochanter due to a tight IT band subluxing/snapping over the greater trochanter
- Sensation of snapping or popping over greater trochanter
- Can reproduce snapping by lying patient on their side and internally and externally rotating the leg (log rolling)
- Workup: none
- Treatment: rest, ice, NSAIDs, PT, US-guided corticosteroid injection if bursitis

Greater Trochanteric Bursitis

- AKA greater trochanteric pain syndrome
- AKA subgluteus maximus bursitis
- True greater trochanteric bursitis is inflammation of the subgluteus maximus bursa located at the greater trochanter, just deep to the gluteus maximus muscle, and just superficial to the gluteus medius tendon as it inserts onto greater trochanter
    - Essentially the tiny bursa right between the glut max and glut med at the greater trochanter
- Important distinction, because there are also bursae located beneath the gluteus medius and gluteus minimus tendons
- **Important point:** while greater trochanteric pain syndrome is very common, in contrast to this true, actual greater trochanteric *bursitis* is rare. It is far more likely that your

patient has gluteus medius tendonitis/tendonopathy than an actual distended, inflamed bursa. Thus, most palpation-guided greater trochanteric "bursa" injections are actually gluteal tendon corticosteroid injections, which do not promote proper tendon healing.

Greater Trochanteric Bursitis

- Pain in lateral thigh, worse with walking or lying on that side, due to actual subgluteus maximus bursopathy (distended, angry, fluid-filled bursa)
- Due to primarily hip abductor weakness (gluteus medius, TFL)
  - Obesity, deconditioning, stroke, TBI, age
- **Workup:** physical exam (localized pain over greater trochanter)
- **Treatment:** rest, ice, NSAIDs, PT, US-guided corticosteroid injection

Hip Flexor Strain

- Tear of the iliopsoas due to attempting to flex the hip while it is forcefully being extended, or with overly forceful hip flexion (e.g. soccer, kicking, sprinting)
- Pain in proximal groin with resisted hip flexion or with hip extension while palpating the iliopsoas muscle
- **Workup:** xrays to rule out ASIS or AIIS avulsion fracture (ASIS - may occur with sartorious strain or iliopsoas strain; AIIS - rectus femoris strain), US
- **Treatment:** rest, ice, NSAIDS, PT

Hamstring Strain

- Tear of the proximal hamstrings due to eccentric stretching of the muscle against a stronger hip flexion and knee extension force
- Pain at ischial tuberosity with resisted knee flexion, or with hip flexion and knee extension (stretching the hamstrings) while palpating the proximal hamstrings/ischial tuberosity
- Commonly happens as a water-skiing injury
- You might see extensive bruising in the posterior thigh
- **Workup:** xrays to rule out ischial tuberosity avulsion fracture, US
- **Treatment:** rest, ice, NSAIDs, PT

Adductor Strain

- Tearing of the proximal thigh adductors, usually due to an eccentric injury (trying to adduct the thigh while it is being abducted by other, stronger forces)
- Pain in proximal medial thigh with resisted adduction or palpating proximal medial thigh while abducting the leg
- **Workup:** xrays to rule out avulsion fracture at the adductor tubercle

- **Treatment:** rest, ice, NSAIDs, PT

Piriformis Syndrome

- Pain in buttock and posterior thigh due to a tight/swollen/inflamed piriformis muscle impinging upon the sciatic nerve
- The sciatic nerve usually courses underneath (deep to) the piriformis, but in some cases it pierces the piriformis muscle belly, making it more susceptible to undue compression by the piriformis
- Pain and numbness/tingling down the leg with FAIR test
    - Flexion, adduction, internal rotation of thigh
- **Workup:** consider xrays, as other pathology might be causing the pain (e.g. SI joint), US
- **Treatment:** rest, NSAIDs, PT (stretching and strengthening of piriformis and other external rotators), US-guided corticosteroid injection to piriformis, botulinum toxin in refractory cases

Myositis Ossificans

- Heterotopic ossification in an area of muscle, usually due to trauma and hematoma formation in the muscle
    - This hematoma breaks down and leads to HO bone formation
- Usually the quadriceps of young, active males
- Usually self-limiting after about 1 year
- Localized pain, swelling, palpable mass in the muscle
- **Workup:** xrays (after 2-3 weeks), MRI if earlier, US
- **Treatment:** rest, ROM, PT, surgery at 10-12 months of maturity if still symptomatic

Eight chapters down! What a mental workout. You can almost feel the physiatry in your bones!

Chapter 9: Musculoskeletal Medicine
Knee

The Knee

- Hinge joint

- Largest joint in the body

- Hyaline (articular) cartilage (contains type II collagen)

- Collagen
    - Type I: skin and normal tendons
    - Type II: hyaline/articular cartilage
    - Type III: tendonosis tendons
    - Type IV: basement membrane

- The knee performs flexion, extension, internal rotation, external rotation

Knee Bony Anatomy

- Femur and tibia come together to form the bony articulation

- The fibula is lateral and below the actual joint

- Patellofemoral joint is also at play

- **Femur** has medial and lateral condyles from which the MCL and LCL originate and stretch down to attach to the tibial shaft and fibular head, respectively

- **Tibia** also has medial and lateral condyles

- The 4 condyles of the femur and tibia altogether articulate to form the tibiofemoral joint (the knee)

Knee Ligaments

- ACL
    - Starts on femur and runs **antero-infero-medially** to attach onto the tibia
    - **Tenses with knee extension**
    - Limits translation of the tibia in the anterior direction
        - **Prevents the tibia from moving forward**
    - With knee flexion, the tibia will curve under the femur, which will cause the ACL to **pull the femur anteriorly**

- PCL
    - Starts on femur and runs **postero-infero-laterally** to attach onto the tibia
    - **Tenses with knee flexion**
    - **Limits translation of the tibia in the posterior direction**

Knee Ligaments

- **MCL**
  - Extends from medial femoral condyle to medial tibia
  - Prevents valgus deviation of the knee
  - **Its deep fibers attach to the medial meniscus**
  - Thus, when MCL tears, check for medial meniscal tear as well
    - **Beware O'Donoghue's triad of ACL, MCL, medial meniscus tear**
      - "Terrible triad"
- **LCL**
  - Extends from lateral femoral condyle to fibular head
  - Prevents varus deviation of the knee

Neuromuscular Overview

- Your knee flexes, extends, internally rotates, externally rotates
- Let's cover the major muscles and nerves that make this happen

Knee Flexion

- Hamstrings
  - Originate at ischial tuberosity
    - Conjoint tendon houses the semitendinosus and biceps femoris medially
    - Semimembranosus tendon originates laterally
    - Ultimately going down the thigh, the muscles separate out as "MTB" going medially to laterally
  - Semimembranosus, semitendinosus
    - L4, L5, S1, sciatic nerve (tibial division)
  - Biceps femoris
    - L5, S1, sciatic nerve (tibial or fibular division depending on long or short head)
- Sartorius
- Gastrocnemius
  - S1, S2, tibial nerve

Knee Extension

- Quadriceps femoris
  - Rectus femoris, vastus intermedius, vastus medialis (VMO), vastus lateralis
  - L2, L3, L4, femoral nerve

Knee Internal Rotation

- Semimembranosus, semitendinosus
  - L4, L5, S1, sciatic nerve (tibial division)
- Sartorius
- Gracilis
  - L2, L3, L4, obturator nerve
- **S**ay **G**race before **T**ea at the pes anserine (anteromedial tibial attachment for **s**artorius, **g**racilis, semi**t**endinosus)

Knee External Rotation

- Biceps femoris
  - L5, S1, sciatic nerve (tibial or fibular division depending on long or short head)

Unlocking the Knee

- Popliteus muscle

Knee Osteoarthritis

- Degeneration of the articular cartilage of the knee due to wear and tear
- Not an inflammatory primary process
- Gradual onset, progressive vague knee pain and stiffness (<1 hour) that is worse with activity and weight-bearing
- Trauma, obesity, weak muscles of the hip and knee are risk factors
- Workup: xrays (medial compartment narrowing, reactive bony sclerosis, reactive osteophytes, subchondral cysts)
- Treatment: rest, ice, acetaminophen, NSAIDs, PT, corticosteroid/PRP injection, total knee replacement

Tibial Plateau Fracture

- Proximal tibia fracture along the "plateau/apex" of the tibia at the joint
- Usually due to high-energy impact (trauma, falls)
- Pain in knee region with history of trauma/fall/impact
- **Workup:** xrays, CT scan for surgical planning
- **Treatment:**
  - Conservative if minimally displaced, stable (bracing, PWB)
  - ORIF otherwise

Osteochondritis Dissecans

- AVN to an area of bone (typically medial femoral condyle or distal femur) due to repetitive stress to that area, that results in *dissection* (separation) of that piece of bone away from the rest of the bone

- Usually in early teenagers

- Knee pain, knee giving out, effusion

- **Workup:** xrays (may see detached bone fragment), MRI

- **Treatment:** rest and NWB so it can heal; surgery if fragment has already detached

Popliteal Artery Entrapment Syndrome (PAES)

- Popliteal artery of males in their 20s/30s becomes compressed in the popliteal fossa due to a variety of reasons, usually because of abnormal course or abnormal muscle impinging on it

- Lower limb swelling and discomfort with numbness and tingling in the lower limb or foot

- Check for decreased dorsalis pedis pulse with plantar flexion

- **Workup:** arteriogram

- **Treatment:** activity modification if disease is mild; otherwise vascular bypass

ACL Tear

- Tear of the anterior cruciate ligament (ACL), usually from a noncontact cutting type of movement (e.g. football, soccer)

- Remember, the ACL is tense in knee extension, so if the knee is extended while attempting to cut, this places the ACL at greatest tension/risk of tear

- This is the most commonly injured knee ligament in sports

- Associated with O'Donoghue's Triad (ACL/MCL/medial meniscus triple tear)

- Sudden popping sound/sensation, knee pain, swelling +/- hemarthrosis
  - Anterior drawer (tibia translates anteriorly with soft or no distinct endpoint)
  - Lachman is more sensitive test (tibia translates forward with soft or no distinct endpoint)

ACL Tear

- **Workup:** xrays (possible avulsion fracture where the ACL inserts onto the tibia), joint aspiration may reveal blood, MRI, US, arthroscopy

- **Treatment:** rest, ice, PWB, PT; ACL reconstruction if young, athletic, high-demand athlete

- Anticipate 6-12 months of PT before return to play

- Consider Lenox-Hill derotation orthosis for knee bracing

PCL Tear

- Tear of the posterior cruciate ligament (PCL) usually due to striking the knees against the dashboard in a car accident

- Remember, the PCL is most tense when the knee is flexed, such as sitting in a car

- Sudden pop, knee pain, swelling, stiffness
  - Posterior drawer test (tibia translates posteriorly without a distinct endpoint)
  - Sag test (compare both knees and notice that the affected tibia hangs lower than the other)

- **Workup**: xrays to rule out avulsion fracture, MRI, arthroscopy

- **Treatment**: rest, PT; PCL repair if athletic or avulsion fracture is present

MCL Tear

- Tear of the medial collateral ligament (MCL) of the knee, usually due to valgus impact/stress to the knee

- Most common knee ligament torn overall

- Associated with O'Donoghue's Triad (torn ACL/MCL/medial meniscus)

- Medial knee pain with possible swelling
  - Valgus stress test is positive

- **Workup**: xrays for valgus stress radiographs and to rule out epiphyseal fracture, MRI, US

- **Treatment**: rest, ice, NSAIDs, bracing for stability, PT, surgical repair

LCL Tear

- Tear of the lateral collateral ligament (LCL) of the knee, usually due to knee dislocation

- Not common

- Common fibular nerve is nearby, so beware of injury to it

- **Workup**: xrays for varus stress radiographs, and to rule out bony pathology, MRI, US

- **Treatment**: rest, ice, NSAIDs, knee bracing for stability, PT, surgical repair

Meniscal Tear

- Tear of the medial or lateral meniscus (fibrocartilage cushions) of the knee, usually due to degeneration along with OA, or landing from a jump and cutting/twisting the knee/squatting
  - Basically grinding the knee under force will help tear the menisci
  - This is exactly what our physical exam tests for the menisci are trying to do

- Think **MC** Hammer (**m**edial meniscus is **C**-shaped while lateral meniscus is O-shaped)

- Sensation of popping, knee pain, swelling over 24 hours (more gradual than ACL/PCL), locking or catching of the knee when attempting to flex or extend

- Medial or lateral joint line tenderness is the most sensitive test for medial or lateral meniscus injuries, respectively

  - McMurray, Apley Grind, Thessaly, deep squatting and twisting, Bounce Home

Meniscal Tear

- **Workup:** xrays, MRI, MR arthrogram, US

- **Treatment:** rest, ice, acetaminophen, NSAIDs, PT

  - Surgical resection of the meniscus if the injury involves the inner 2/3 portion, as only the outer 1/3 portion is well vascularized

  - Because the inner 2/3 is poorly vascularized, it's not going to heal if you perform surgery on it, so we just take it out

  - Surgical repair is indicated for injuries to the outer 1/3 of the meniscus

Plica

- Redundant fold of synovial tissue of the knee that can become thickened and inflamed, leading to anterior knee pain with locking/catching and buckling

- The plica can become trapped with flexion and extension, leading to locking and catching

- Often it is asymptomatic, but occasionally leads to plica syndrome as above

- **Workup:** xrays, MRI if PFPS symptoms are not improving

- **Treatment:** same as PFPS; surgery to remove plica

Baker Cyst

- Inflammation and fluid collection within the posterior knee bursa between the medial head of the gastrocnemius and semimembranosus

- Palpable mass/swelling/fluid collection

- **Workup:** MRI, US (use doppler to rule out DVT/aneurysm)

- **Treatment:** avoid aggravating factors, PT, aspiration and steroid injection, surgical excision

Pes Anserine Bursitis

- Tendons of the sartorius, gracilis, and semitendinosus insert together onto the pes anserine of the anteromedial tibia

- The pes anserine bursa is right in there

- May become inflamed and swollen due to general knee overuse, tight/weak muscles

- **Workup:** none/MRI, US

- **Treatment:** rest, ice, NSAIDs, US-guided aspiration and steroid injection, surgical excision

Prepatellar Bursitis

- Pain in the anterior bursa between the patella and the skin, usually due to excessive friction or kneeling on the patella (Housemaid's Knee)

- **Workup:** none/MRI, US

- **Treatment:** rest, ice, NSAIDs, knee pads, PT, US-guided aspiration and steroid injection

Superficial and Deep Infrapatellar Bursitis

- Pain in the anterior knee at the patellar tendon due to excessive kneeling on the patellar tendons

- Superficial infrapatellar bursa is just superficial to the patellar tendon

- Deep infrapatellar bursa is just deep to the patellar tendon

- The patellar tendon itself is inferior (infra) to the patella, hence the name

- **Workup:** none/MRI, US

- **Treatment:** rest, ice, NSAIDs, knee pads, PT, US-guided aspiration and steroid injection

Patellofemoral Pain Syndrome (PFPS)

- Anterior knee pain due to improper tracking of the patella along the distal femur, usually secondary to quadriceps weakness/imbalance

- This leads to synovitis around the patella, which is painful

- Common in runners

- Typically pain occurs with stair climbing/descending, running downhill
  - Knee stiffness after prolonged sitting is common

- **Workup:** xrays to assess patellofemoral contours and patella height/position

- **Treatment:** relative rest, ice, NSAIDs, PT (IT band and vastus lateralis stretching, VMO and hip girdle strengthening), patellar knee sleeve with patellar cutout, kinesiotaping for proper tracking of the patella; surgery if all the above fail after 6 months

Chondromalacia Patella

- Generally a sequela of patellofemoral pain syndrome

- Patellar cartilage degenerates and becomes soft due to improper tracking

- Anterior knee pain, similar to PFPS

- **Workup:** xrays as in PFPS, MRI, arthroscopy

- **Treatment:** same as PFPS

Patellar Tendonitis

- Pain in the patellar tendon, usually with jumping activities (e.g. basketball, volleyball), usually in the proximal patellar tendon (inferior pole of patella)

- Overuse of the patellar tendon leads to tendonitis, or tendonosis if chronic

- **Workup:** xrays to examine patellofemoral anatomy, MRI, US

- **Treatment:** same as PFPS, US-guided PRP or tendon scraping

Quadriceps Tendonitis

- Pain in the anterior knee over the quadriceps tendon as it inserts onto the patella, usually due to inflammation of the quad tendon from overuse (e.g. jumping in basketball/volleyball)

- Pain with resisted knee extension

- **Workup:** xrays to evaluate patellofemoral contour/anatomy, MRI, US

- **Treatment:** rest, ice, NSAIDs, PT

Popliteus Tendonitis

- Pain in lateral knee due to popliteus tendon inflammation (overuse), usually during downhill running or skiing

- Pain on palpation of lateral knee

- Popliteus function is to unlock the knee

- **Workup:** none; US may reveal popliteus tendon structural abnormalities as it originates from lateral femoral condyle and inserts onto the posterior tibia)

- **Treatment:** rest, ice, NSAIDs, PT

IT Band Syndrome

- Painful anterior/lateral knee pain, worse after activity (e.g. long distance running), due to excessive snapping or friction of the IT band over the lateral femoral condyle on its way down to attach to Gerdy's tubercle on the lateral tibia

- IT band is an extension of the TFL

- IT band syndrome occurs generally due to weakness and tightness of the TFL, IT band, gluteus medius (hip girdle weakness)

- Ober test is positive

- Pain over lateral femoral condyle with flexion and extension while palpating distal IT band/Gerdy's tubercle

- **Workup:** none/xrays to rule out avulsion fracture

- **Treatment:** rest, ice, NSAIDs, PT for hip girdle stretching and strengthening, US-guided corticosteroid injection to distal IT band

Do you feel it? It's the fear of the board exam as your knowledge grows stronger by the day! The confusing ligaments of the knee trip up most doctors. Little does the exam know that the knee now is your strong point!

Chapter 10: Musculoskeletal Medicine
Lower Leg and Ankle

The Lower Leg Region

- Tibia and fibula are the two bones, connected by an interosseous membrane
- Tibia is the primary weight-bearing bone
  - Hence, shin splints, stress fractures, acute fractures tend to happen to the tibia
- Contains 4 compartments
  - Anterior compartment (most common place for compartment syndrome)
  - Lateral compartment
  - Superficial posterior compartment
  - Deep posterior compartment
- The muscles originating in this region provide neuromuscular control to the ankle

Compartments of the Lower Leg

- **Anterior**
  - Contains dorsiflexors and toe extensors
  - Tibialis anterior (TA), extensor hallucis longus (EHL), extensor digitorum longus (EDL), fibularis tertius, anterior tibial artery (becomes dorsalis pedis artery in the ankle), deep fibular nerve
- **Lateral**
  - Contains plantar flexors and evertors
  - Fibularis longus, fibularis brevis, superficial fibular nerve
- **Superficial posterior**
  - Contains plantar flexors
  - Gastrocnemius, soleus, plantaris
- **Deep posterior**
  - Contains invertors and toe flexors
  - Tibialis posterior (TP), flexor digitorum longus (FDL), flexor hallucis longus (FHL), posterior tibial artery, tibial nerve
    - All pass through the tarsal tunnel to enter the plantar surface of the foot

The Ankle + Bony Anatomy

- Tibiotalar joint is the point of transition from lower leg to ankle
  - It's what we think of when we think "ankle joint" = tibiotalar joint
- The medial part of the tibia extends down and becomes the medial malleolus
  - The tarsal tunnel wraps around the posterior/inferior part of the medial malleolus to enter the foot

- The lateral part of the fibula extends down *even lower* and becomes the lateral malleolus
    - The fibularis tendons wrap around the posterior/inferior part of the lateral malleolus to enter the foot
- The calcaneus (heel bone) sits below the talus, and the navicular sits medially in front of the calcaneus
- *A ton of ligaments* holds all these bones together

Ankle Ligaments

- ATFL (anterior talofibular ligament)
    - Resists anterior translation of the talus/foot
    - Most commonly injured ankle ligament (lateral ankle sprains)
- CFL (calcaneofibular ligament)
    - 2nd ligament to be injured in a lateral ankle sprain
    - Sits near the fibularis longus and brevis tendons as they wrap around the lateral malleolus
- PTFL (posterior talofibular ligament)
- Deltoid ligament
    - Medial ankle stabilizer
    - Not commonly injured (very strong)
- Tibiofibular syndesmosis
    - Anterior/posterior tibiofibular ligaments
    - Interosseous ligament

Neuromuscular Overview of the Ankle

- Your ankle plantarflexes, dorsiflexes, inverts, everts, pronates, supinates
- Let's go over the major muscles and nerves that make this happen

Ankle Plantarflexion

- Gastrocnemius
    - S1, S2, tibial nerve
- Soleus
    - S1, S2, tibial nerve
- Plantaris
- Tibialis posterior
    - L5, S1, tibial nerve
- FHL, FDL, fibularis longus, fibularis brevis also contribute

Ankle Dorsiflexion

- Tibialis anterior
  - L4, L5, deep fibular nerve
- Fibularis tertius
  - L5, S1, deep fibular nerve
- EHL and EDL also contribute

Ankle Inversion

- Tibialis posterior
  - L5, S1, tibial nerve
- Tibialis anterior
  - L4, L5, deep fibular nerve

Ankle Eversion

- Fibularis longus and brevis
  - L5, S1, superficial fibular nerve
- Fibularis tertius
  - L5, S1, deep fibular nerve

Ankle Pronation and Supination

- Pronation: eversion, dorsiflexion, external rotation of the tibia
- Supination: inversion, plantarflexion, internal rotation of the tibia

Maisonneuve Fracture

- A complication of a high ankle sprain; essentially a proximal fibular fracture due to a really bad high ankle sprain (rupture of the tibiofibular syndesmosis)
- The syndesmosis splits, and the split ultimately extends all the way up until it causes a proximal fibular fracture
- **Workup:** xrays
- **Treatment:** generally orthopedic referral

Shin Splints (Medial Tibial Stress Syndrome)

- Medial shin pain due to excessive overload of the tibia over time, including microtears at the muscle-periosteum interface (traction periostitis)
- This usually occurs due to excessive long distance running

- ○ Squeezing the medial and lateral sides of the tibia together (tibial squeeze) reproduces the pain along the entire length (or even just a small portion) of the tibia
- **Workup:** xrays (evaluate for stress fracture), MRI
- **Treatment:** shoe orthotics, softer running surface, correct running gait (overpronation is common training error), reduce mileage, relative rest, PT, NSAIDs, ice, surgery (fasciotomy)

Tibial Stress Fracture

- Can be the result of untreated shin splints, or present similarly
- Actual microfracture of the tibia due to overuse (excessive running)
- Too much, too far, too fast
- **Workup:** xrays, MRI (bone marrow edema)
- **Treatment:** similar to shin splints.
    - ○ Relative rest (NWB progressing to WB if pain with normal ambulation)
    - ○ Acetaminophen, ice
    - ○ Ultimately PT, reintroduce running, correct gait mechanics, strengthen hip girdle
    - ○ Re-image to follow fracture healing before elevating activity (running again)
    - ○ Surgery if fracture is big, or involves the anterior cortex

Talus Fracture

- Fracture of the bone that articulates with the tibia (and fibula, navicular, calcaneus) to form the ankle joint, usually due to forced dorsiflexion with an axial load applied upward (from the plantar surface)
- Can fracture the talar head, neck, and body (AKA dome)
- Talar body (AKA dome) fractures have a greater risk of AVN
- **Workup:** xrays, MRI
- **Treatment:** NWB if nondisplaced and low risk for AVN; ORIF otherwise

Calcaneus Fracture

- Most common foot fracture, due to traumatic axial load (e.g. a long fall)
- Pain, bruising, swelling, disfigurement at heels
- **Workup:** xrays
- **Treatment:** cast and NWB if stress fracture or very small fracture; otherwise ORIF

Sever's Disease

- Posterior heel pain in children (usually athletes) due to excessive overuse of the gastroc pulling on the calcaneus, resulting in calcaneal apophysitis

- **Workup:** xrays/MRI sometimes indicated to rule out other causes of heel pain

- **Treatment:** usually self-limiting; calf stretches, ice, NSAIDs, relative rest

Syndesmosis Injury / High Ankle Sprain

- Injury of the tibiofibular syndesmosis (interosseous membrane) due to excessive external rotation forces (common football injury)
  - The talus pushes into the fibula, separating the fibula away from the tibia, tearing the ligaments holding them together

- Pain in lower leg with swelling

- Often the AITFL and PTFL are torn as well

- Sometimes the split of the interosseous membrane extends upward high enough into the leg to cause a Maisonneuve fracture (proximal fibula fracture)

- Squeeze test is positive (squeezing tibia and fibula together elicits pain)

- **Workup:** xrays, MRI if bones look normal and still suspect high ankle sprain

- **Treatment:** NWB in CAM boot for 3 weeks; surgery especially if bony instability

Lateral Ankle Sprain

- Injury of the ATFL/CFL/PTFL due to excessive inversion forces on the ankle
  - Rolling your ankle inward
  - This is the most common type and mechanism of ankle sprain

- The order of ligaments torn is typically: ATFL → CFL → PTFL

- Grade 1 sprain: partially torn ATFL, intact CFL

- Grade 2 sprain: fully torn ATFL, partially torn CFL

- Grade 3 sprain: fully torn ATFL, fully torn CFL

- Anterior drawer (ATFL) and talar tilt (CFL) tests are often positive

- Beware of fibularis longus/brevis tendon injury as well!

- **Workup:** xrays with stress views (exams above), MRI, US

- **Treatment:** rest, ice, compression, elevation, NSAIDs, bracing to immobilize, PT; surgical repair of ligaments indicated if high-level athlete or failed conservative care

Medial Ankle Sprain

- Tear of the deltoid ligament at the medial aspect of the ankle due to excessive eversion forces, leading to medial ankle pain and swelling

- Not nearly as common as lateral ankle sprains, due to the strength of the ligaments involved

- The deltoid ligament is actually:
  - Anterior tibiotalar ligament, posterior tibiotalar ligament, tibionavicular ligament, tibiocalcaneal ligament

- **Workup:** xrays, MRI

- **Treatment:** rest, ice, NSAIDs, brace immobilization for several weeks, PT; surgical repair

Tarsal Tunnel Syndrome

- Tarsal Tunnel: region behind the medial malleolus, involving structures that pass underneath the flexor retinaculum and sometimes become compressed by it
  - Tibial nerve
  - Tibial artery
  - Tibial vein
  - Tibialis posterior (TP)
  - Flexor digitorum longus (FDL)
  - Flexor hallucis longus (FHL)

- Pain, numbness, tingling, foot weakness, due to tight compression of the tibial nerve underneath the flexor retinaculum

- **Workup:** xrays, MRI, EMG, US

- **Treatment:** PT, NSAIDs, US-guided steroid injection, surgical release

Ankle Bursitis

- Inflammation of fluid-filled synovial fluid sac near the ankle

- Usually due to excessive friction forces (e.g. high heels)
  - The visible soft tissue swelling you see is called a Haglund deformity AKA "pump bump"

- Retrocalcaneal bursa: just posterior to the calcaneus (between calcaneus and achilles tendon)

- Retroachilles bursa: between achilles tendon and skin

- Palpable soft tissue mass on exam

- **Workup:** none

- **Treatment:** don't wear high heels or shoes that irritate the posterior heel; US-guided steroid injection; surgical removal

Acute Compartment Syndrome (ACS) of the Leg

- Emergency condition in which the pressure within a leg compartment rises to incredibly high levels, such that venous return is disrupted, and all the tissues within the compartment may become ischemic, leading to necrosis
    - This includes muscles and nerves
- Blood can pump in, but it can't pump out
- Usually due to trauma, fracture
- Usually takes place in the **anterior compartment**
- Pain, paresthesias, paralysis
    - Extreme, **out of normal proportion pain to stretching the muscles of that compartment**
- If allowed to progress, foot drop may be a chronic sequela
- **Workup:** compartment pressure testing (manometry)
- **Treatment:** emergent fasciotomy

Chronic Exertional Compartment Syndrome

- Chronic condition of temporarily raised intracompartmental pressure during exercise
- Symptoms include pain, paresthesias, weakness, worse as the exercise continues or increases in intensity, improved or resolved by rest
- **Workup:** compartment manometry before and after exercise to demonstrate pressure increase; consider xrays/MRI to rule out shin splints, stress fractures, etc.
- **Treatment:** fasciotomy

Tibialis Anterior Tendon Injury

- Injury of the tibialis anterior tendon (dorsiflexor and inverter) due to overuse (tenosynovitis) or rupture (eccentric overload)
- Tenosynovitis may be due to excessive pressure from the extensor retinaculum as the TA tendon passes underneath it in the anterior ankle
- Foot slap may be audible/visible
- Pain with resisted dorsiflexion or passive plantarflexion with palpation of tendon
- **Workup:** none/MRI/US
- **Treatment:** rest, ice, NSAIDs, PT, US-guided steroid/PRP, surgery

Tibialis Posterior Tendon Injury

- Injury and degeneration of the tibialis posterior tendon (plantarflexor and invertor) due to repetitive overuse forces on the muscle/tendon unit
    - Gait abnormalities increase risk for this (excessive pronation)

- ○ Can also occur with medial ankle sprains (stretch injury)
- Medial retromalleolar pain and swelling, worse with resisted inversion and plantarflexion
- Positive Too Many Toes sign
- **Workup:** none/US/MRI
- **Treatment:** rest, ice, NSAIDs, orthotics, correct gait and running mechanics, US-guided corticosteroid/PRP injection; surgical intervention

Flexor Hallucis Longus Injury

- Overuse injury of the FHL (the long big toe flexor) often due to dancing (dancer's tendonitis), actions involving a lot of big toe flexion against resistance
- Pain with resisted big toe flexion or passive extension; pain may occur behind medial malleolus as tendon wraps around in the tarsal tunnel
- **Workup:** none/MRI/US
- **Treatment:** rest, ice, NSAIDs, PT

Fibularis Tendon Injury

- Injury of the fibularis longus and/or brevis, often due to overuse eversion activity (overpronation, sports) or as a result of a bad lateral ankle sprain, stretching the tendons and tearing them
- Pain with resisted plantarflexion and eversion or passive dorsiflexion and inversion
- **Workup:** xray if concerned about bones after trauma, MRI, US
- **Treatment:** rest, ice, NSAIDs, PT, US-guided steroid/PRP, surgical repair

Achilles Tendon Injury

- Pain in the posterior heel over the achilles tendon and calcaneus due to overuse (repetitive eccentric overload) of the tendon, leading to inflammation and degeneration of the tendon
- Improper healing of the tendon may occur, leading to tendonosis
- Poor vascularity in the distal 2-6 cm of the tendon predisposes to tears
- Age, overtraining, overpronation, tight achilles tendons are all risk factors
- Achilles tendon rupture is usually due to huge eccentric forces (trauma, sports) rupturing the tendon (sudden pop, swelling, bruising, pain)
- Thompson test is positive in acute ruptures
- **Workup:** none/MRI/US
- **Treatment:** RICE, PT (heavy slow resistance), US-guided PRP; consider plantarflexion bracing progressing to neutral vs. surgical repair for ruptures

Ten of twenty-five chapters down! But you are more than ten twenty-fifths of a physiatrist!

Chapter 11: Musculoskeletal Medicine
Foot

The Foot

- The foot is made up of 7 tarsal bones
  - Calcaneus (heel bone; achilles attaches here)
  - Talus (sits on top of calcaneus and articulates with tibia, fibula)
  - Navicular (medial side of foot, in front of talus)
  - Cuboid (lateral side of foot, in front of talus)
  - Medial, intermediate, and lateral cuneiforms
- Metatarsals for each digit
- Phalanges for each digit
- 2 sesamoid bones sit on the plantar side of the first metatarsal head
- Everything is held together by ligaments with tendons pulling on various bones
- We talked about ankle motion during the last section
  - Plantarflexion, dorsiflexion, inversion, eversion, pronation, supination
- The major foot actions are to flex, extend, abduct, adduct the toes

Ligaments of the Foot

- Lisfranc ligament: attaches the medial cuneiform to the 2nd metatarsal
  - Common ligament sprain in athletics (football)
- Transverse metatarsal ligament: strings together the metatarsal heads by running across the anterior surface of all of them
- Calcaneonavicular "spring" ligament: connects these two bones; maintains the medial longitudinal arch of the foot
  - Medial longitudinal arch: the arch shape of the medial foot, formed by the bones and pulled into position by the ligaments and tendons of the foot and ankle
  - Pes planus: flat arches
  - Pes cavus: high arch (arches as big as a cave!)

Neuromuscular Overview of the Foot

- Your foot flexes, extends, adducts, and abducts the toes
- If these intrinsic foot muscles have compromised neurologic control, then clawing of the toes may occur due to intrinsic muscle weakness
  - Charcot-Marie-Tooth (CMT) disease
- Let's go over the major muscles and nerves that make this happen

Toe Flexion

- Flexor digitorum longus (FDL)
  - L5, S1, tibial nerve
- Flexor hallucis longus (FHL)
  - L5, S1, tibial nerve
- Flexor hallucis brevis (FHB)
  - S1, S2, tibial nerve → medial plantar nerve

Toe Extension

- Extensor digitorum longus (EDL)
  - L4, L5, deep fibular nerve
- Extensor digitorum brevis (EDB)
  - L4, L5, S1, deep fibular nerve
- Extensor hallucis longus (EHL)
  - L4, L5, S1, deep fibular nerve

Toe Adduction

- Adductor hallucis
  - S1, S2, tibial nerve → lateral plantar nerve
- Palmar interossei (3)
  - S2, S3, tibial nerve → lateral plantar nerve

Toe Abduction

- Abductor hallucis
  - S1, S2, tibial nerve → medial plantar nerve
- Dorsal interossei (4)
  - S2, S3, tibial nerve → lateral plantar nerve
- Abductor digiti quinti pedis (ADQP)
  - S1, S2, tibial nerve → inferior calcaneal nerve (or LPN depending on whom you ask)

Charcot Foot/Joint

- This is an arthritic, likely deformed joint due to poor sensation and proprioception of the foot
- Poor muscular control, sensation, and proprioception mean you cannot protect the joint properly when walking
- The joint gets beat up over time and degenerates

- Typically caused by diabetes → neuropathy
- **Workup:** history, physical exam, xrays (joint space narrowing, osteophytes, disfigurement), EMG/NCS potentially
- **Treatment:** PT, OT, orthotics, assistive devices

March Fracture

- Pain and swelling in the distal foot due to a metatarsal stress fracture due to e.g. marching; excessive bone stress
- **Workup:** xrays, MRI
- **Treatment:** rest, ice, immobilization brace, acetaminophen, surgery (ORIF) if displacement or on 5th metatarsal

Jones Fracture

- Pain and swelling in the distal foot due to a fracture across the base of the 5th metatarsal, usually due a forceful inversion or adduction injury
- **Workup:** xrays, MRI
- **Treatment:** NWB vs. surgery depending on type and severity

Nutcracker Fracture

- Cuboid fracture due to trauma
- Pain and swelling in foot over the cuboid
- Imagine a nutcracker cracking a cube
- **Workup:** xrays, MRI
- **Treatment:** surgery

Hallux Rigidus

- 1st MTP joint arthritis due to wear and tear
- Pain, stiffness of big toe
- **Workup:** xrays (joint space narrowing, osteophytes)
- **Treatment:** high/wide toe box shoes, comfortable orthotics, acetaminophen/NSAIDs; surgery (joint debridement)

Hallux Valgus and Bunions

- Lateral deviation of the big toe (excessive adduction), causing a painful medial 1st MTP bump or prominence (bunion)
- Usually due to genetics or too narrow shoes
- **Workup:** none/xrays

- **Treatment:** rest, ice, acetaminophen/NSAIDs, comfortable orthotics, wide toe box shoes; surgical bunionectomy

Hammer Toe

- MTP extension, **PIP flexion**, DIP extension usually due to shoes being too small (not long enough toe box)
- **Workup:** xrays
- **Treatment:** correct the footwear (purchase larger shoes with higher toe box), ROM of toes

Mallet Toe

- MTP normal, PIP normal, **DIP flexion** usually due to wearing shoes that are too small/tight, or trauma
- **Workup:** xrays (rule out extensor tendon avulsion fracture)
- **Treatment:** foot orthotics, larger shoes with higher toe box, trim the callus on the toe; surgical flexor tenotomy

Claw Toe

- MTP extension, **PIP flexion, DIP flexion** due to intrinsic foot muscle weakness
- Usually due to neurologic disease (DM2, CMT)
- **Workup:** xrays, often discovered during EMG for other reasons
- **Treatment:** soft orthotics, high toe box shoes; surgery to correct deformity

1st Metatarsophalangeal Joint Sprain (MTP)

- AKA Turf Toe
- Sprain of the joint capsule and ligaments of the 1st MTP joint, usually due to cutting on a hard surface with flexible shoes, leading to a hyperextension injury of the 1st MTP joint
- Pain is reproduced with extending the 1st MTP
- **Workup:** xrays
- **Treatment:** rest, ice, NSAIDs, firm shoes, metatarsal splinting, orthotics

Lisfranc Joint Injury

- Injury/tear of the lisfranc ligament which connects the medial cuneiform bone with the 2nd metatarsal; this is what we call a tarsometatarsal joint
- Usually due to athletic trauma (football)
- Dorsal foot pain in the region of that tarsometatarsal joint

- Pain is reproduced with fixing the ankle in place and shearing the foot bones away from the ankle
- **Workup:** xrays, MRI
- **Treatment:** rest, NWB for several weeks; ORIF if unstable

Morton Neuroma

- Interdigital benign growth of nerve tissue due to repetitive microtrauma to the interdigital nerve, usually the nerve between the 3rd and 4th metatarsals
- Pain radiating between two metatarsals, dysesthesias, paresthesias
- Positive Morton click on exam
- **Workup:** none/MRI/US
- **Treatment:** comfortable orthotics, wide toe box shoes, metatarsal pads, US-guided corticosteroid injection; surgical removal

Plantar fasciitis

- Pulling, tension-like pain at the medial heel and medial arch of foot, worst upon awakening and taking first steps out of bed, improving with continued walking
- Due to plantar fascia inflammation
  - HLA-B27, seronegative spondyloarthropathy, calcaneal bone spur associations
  - Pes cavus, pes planus, tight achilles tendon are other risk factors
- Pain reproducible with big toe extension while palpating the medial plantar heel
- **Workup:** none/xrays/MRI
- **Treatment:** plantar fascia stretching, nighttime dorsiflexion splints, NSAIDs, orthotics, US-guided corticosteroid injection; surgical plantar fascia release

Keep your head up. Musculoskeletal medicine is complex. Nobody learns it in a day! Congrats on making it head to toe. Now let's finish with the spine.

Chapter 12: Musculoskeletal Medicine
Spine

The Spine

- Interconnecting column of bones, ligaments, discs, and nervous tissue that serves as the axial foundation of the body

- All joints connect in some way to the spine

- If your spine is dysfunctional, other joints can become dysfunctional → pain

- If other joints are dysfunctional, your spine can become dysfunctional → pain

- 7 cervical vertebrae (C1-C7)

- 12 thoracic vertebrae (T1-T12)

- 5 lumbar vertebrae (L1-L5)

- 5 sacral vertebrae fused into 1 sacrum

- Coccyx

The Spine

- Your spine flexes, extends, twists, and laterally bends

- It also has natural curves in the sagittal plane
    - Cervical spine → natural lordosis
    - Thoracic spine → natural kyphosis
    - Lumbar spine → natural lordosis
    - Sacral spine → natural kyphosis

- Typically injury to the spine and its contents occur with trauma (e.g. hyperextension), infection, infarction, spondylosis (degenerative cascade)

- The vertebrae are connected at the vertebral endplate-disc-endplate joint and the 2 facet joints off to the side at each level

- Let's discuss spine anatomy

"Typical" Vertebra

- A typical vertebra will have a vertebral body, pedicles, transverse processes, superior and inferior articular processes, laminae, spinous process, and central canal

- Where the SAPs and IAPs join with other vertebrae above and below, these spots are called facet joints

- As we age, our intervertebral discs degenerate, leading to more weight being borne by the facet joints → increased facet arthritis

- Let's draw this out to appreciate it a little better

Cervical Vertebrae

- C1 is also called Atlas
  - Essentially just a big ring of bone for the skull to sit on
- C2 is also called Axis
  - Axis' vertebral body has a dens (AKA odontoid process) poking upward
- The atlantooccipital joint joins Atlas to the occiput (skull)
- The atlantoaxial joint is the C1-C2 joint
- C2-C6 have bifid spinous processes
- C7 is called "vertebra prominens" because it has a very prominent spinous process
- 50% of cervical flexion/extension occurs at atlantooccipital joint
- 50% of cervical rotation occurs at atlantoaxial joint
- C3-C7 have uncinate processes (basically raised edges of the VB) that degenerate over time to become uncovertebral joints

Thoracic Vertebrae

- Everything that a typical vertebra is, except thoracic vertebrae also have joints directly on the VBs for the ribs to attach onto
- The rib attachments are what define a thoracic vertebra

Lumbar Vertebrae

- These vertebrae have the largest VBs, because they are bearing the most weight
- In fact, VB size increases the further inferior you go down the spine
- We normally have 5 lumbar vertebrae (L1-L5), but some individuals have an L6 vertebra, or they only have L1-L4
  - This is called transitional anatomy
  - Lumbarization of the sacrum results when the first sacral bone fails to fuse with the rest of the sacrum, leading to a floating vertebra above the sacrum, below the lumbar spine, and so it is essentially now an L6 vertebra
  - Sacralization of the lumbar spine results when the L5 vertebra fuses with the sacrum, essentially giving you a longer sacrum and shorter lumbar spine (L1-L4)
- Transitional anatomy does not necessarily cause pain or pathology; it is considered a normal variant
- It has implications when trying to choose the correct target for an interventional spine procedure

Sacrum

- The sacrum is actually just 5 fused vertebrae

- It is a big, broad bone that has its own neuroforamina for the S1-S5 nerve roots to exit and innervate their myotomes/dermatomes

Vertebral Body Endplate and Intervertebral Disc

- The vertebral endplate is the flat part of the VB that touches the intervertebral disc
- The intervertebral disc is the squishy jelly donut that sits between VBs to provide axial cushioning; it is comprised of the nucleus pulposus and annulus fibrosus
- The NP is made up of water, type II collagen, and other materials
  - As we age we lose nucleus pulposus water content while fibrous tissue increases
    - This makes the discs darker on T2 MRI as they lose water
  - The nucleus pulposus has no nerve supply, and, thus, cannot be a source of pain
- The annulus fibrosus contains type I collagen

Facet Joints

- AKA zygapophyseal joints
- These are true joints
  - They have cartilage and a joint capsule
- They bear more weight as you go down the spine
- Orientation of facet joints is coronal all the way down, until L1, at which point they are sagittal progressing back to coronal
- Facet joints are innervated by the **medial branches** of the dorsal rami
- In the cervical spine, a given facet joint is innervated by the same numbers as its VBs
  - E.g. the C4-C5 facet is innervated by the C4 and C5 medial branches
- In the lumbar spine, a given facet joint is innervated by that level and the level above
  - E.g. the L3-L4 facet is innervated by the L2 and L3 medial branches

Spinal Ligaments

- **Anterior longitudinal ligament (ALL)**
  - Runs vertically along the anterior VBs to limit extension forces
- **Posterior longitudinal ligament (PLL)**
  - Runs vertically along the posterior VBs to limit flexion forces
- **Ligamentum flavum**
  - Runs vertically in the posterior spine from lamina to lamina
  - Epidural steroid injections pierce the ligamentum flavum to enter the epidural space
- **Supraspinous ligament**
  - Runs vertically to connect spinous process to spinous process

- Above C7 it continues as the ligamentum nuchae

- **Interspinous ligament**
  - Similar to supraspinous ligament, except this is more interiorly placed

Innervations of the Spine

- Nucleus pulposus: lacks innervation

- Annulus fibrosus: ventral rami (anterior), sinuvertebral nerves (posterior)

- Vertebral body: sinuvertebral nerves

- Back muscles, spinal erectors: dorsal primary rami

- Cervical facets: "that level" innervation; e.g. C3-C4 facet = C3, C4 medial branches

- Lumbar facets: "that level + above"; e.g. L4-L5 facet = L3, L4 medial branches

Muscles of the Spine

- Trapezius and latissimus dorsi (superficial)
  - Pull scapula superiorly and medially / adduct and internally rotate humerus

- Splenius capitis/cervicis (superficial)
  - Spinal extension, lateral flexion, ipsilateral rotation

- Spinal erectors (deep) [iliocostalis, longissimus, spinalis, semispinalis, multifidus]
  - Spinal extension

- Many of these muscles become important in myofascial pain and spasticity/dystonia, and thus are high-yield targets for botulinum toxin

Bone Disorders of the Spine

- Some fractures of the spine are covered in the Spinal Cord Injury section

- The rest we will discuss here

Vertebral Body Compression/Burst Fracture

- Crush forces that cause anterior wedging of the VB, usually at the thoracolumbar junction due to trauma/fall, in an osteoporotic patient

- Surgery is indicated in cases of severe, intractable pain, unstable spine, vertebral body height loss greater than 50%, or in the setting of neurologic compromise

- Spine is unstable if the middle column is damaged, or any 2 columns
  - Anterior column = ALL → anterior 2/3 of VB and annulus
  - Middle column = posterior 1/3 of VB and annulus → PLL
  - Posterior column = ligamentum flavum → spinous process

- **Workup:** xrays, CT, MRI (anterior wedging in affected VB)

- **Treatment:** bracing (CASH/Jewett) for comfort and stability; PT; pain control; vertebroplasty/balloon kyphoplasty (though not really effective)

Spinal Stenosis

- Narrowing of the central spinal canal that leads to compression of the neural structures within (spinal cord and nerve roots)
    - Typically lumbar region is affected
    - Narrowing typically due to degenerative spondylosis cascade, disc-osteophyte complexes, etc.
    - This can cause myelopathy or radiculopathy
    - It can also cause "neurogenic claudication", which is different from vascular claudication

- **Neurogenic claudication**
    - Leg or buttock pain, weakness, "leg heaviness" with activity, especially activities that involve spinal extension, which narrows the spinal canal (prolonged standing, walking, walking downhill, standing)
    - Symptoms relieved by spinal flexion (leaning forward on shopping cart, walking uphill, biking), as this opens the spinal canal up and relieves pressure on the neural contents within

Spinal Stenosis

- This differs from vascular claudication, because vascular claudication will be **worse** with walking uphill and biking, and will show skin changes related to poor vasculature (thin, shiny, hairless skin with diminished/absent pulses)

- **Workup:** xrays, CT, CT myelogram, MRI (VB disc herniation-osteophyte complexes, ligamentum flavum hypertrophy, which narrow the central canal)

- **Treatment:** PT with directional preference assessment, surgical decompression (injections don't work)

Spondylosis

- Spondylosis, or chronic "wear and tear" degenerative changes in the spine, occurs via a certain model, progressing in 3 stages

- **Dysfunction**
    - Poor posture, biomechanics, cartilage degradation, all contribute to dysfunctional joints that move poorly and grind bone against bone

- **Instability**
    - All this grinding and breaking down of normal joints causes things to slip and slide
    - Herniated discs can occur in this stage with annulus tears

- **Stability**

- ○ Fibrosis, osteophyte growth, bony changes cause bone to approximate closer to bone and for things to stabilize in a stiff, arthritic manner
- Joint space decreases, osteophytes grow, and the spinal cord and/or nerve roots can become entrapped by stenotic spinal areas (degenerative spinal stenosis)

Spondylolisthesis

- The slipping of one VB in relation to the VB below, usually due to a pars interarticularis fracture (neck of the scottie dog fracture)
  - ○ This etiology is called **isthmic** and is the most common cause
- Usually this is an *anterior* slipping (anterior translation) of one VB over the VB below
  - ○ Anterolisthesis vs. retrolisthesis
- Degenerative spondylolisthesis is also common, especially in adults
  - ○ Slippage occurs due to standard wear and tear of age, insufficiency of bony junctions

Spondylolisthesis

- Grade 0 = normal
- Grade 1 = 1-25% displacement when comparing the two anterior VB surfaces
- Grade 2 = 26-50%
- Grade 3 = 51-75%
- Grade 4 = 76-100%
- Patient has low back pain worse with any general movement of the spine
- **Workup:** xrays (flexion/extension films to check for instability), MRI
- **Treatment:** relative rest, PT for Grade 1, 2, asymptomatic grade 3; surgery for Grade 4, 5

Spondylolysis

- "Vertebrae fracture" usually due to excessive hyperextension forces, resulting in a pars interarticularis defect (the fracture)
  - ○ Pars = neck of the scottie dog
  - ○ The pars is the spot on the lamina that lies right between the SAP and IAP
- Patient has focal low back pain, worse with extension
- **Workup:** oblique xrays (pars fracture), MRI
- **Treatment:** PT if stable; surgery if unstable with spondylolisthesis

Facet Joint Arthropathy

- Degeneration of the articular cartilage of the facet joint, with joint space narrowing, leading to other arthritic changes such as osteophyte formation, and causing paraspinal back pain, worse with extension and twisting maneuvers

- Pain is in a referred distribution, usually a broad area of skin over that facet joint

- **Workup:** xray, CT, MRI (MRI useful for injection planning)

- **Treatment:** PT, pain medications, facet joint steroid injection, 2 medial branch blocks followed by radiofrequency ablation (RFA) of medial branches

Sacroiliac Joint (SI joint) Dysfunction/Arthritis

- Difficult-to-diagnose pain syndrome involving either hypermobility or hypomobility of the SI joint (space between sacrum and ileum); typically low back/upper buttock pain worse with transitional movements (sit → stand)

- +FABERE, Gaenslen, Sacral compression test, Yeoman, Gillet, Seated flexion test

- You want a high number of positive "SI joint maneuvers" above

- **Workup:** xrays (joint space narrowing, osteophytes), CT, MRI
    - Remember: bilateral sacroiliitis is the hallmark of ankylosing spondylitis (AS)

- **Treatment:** PT, pain medications, fluoroscopic or US-guided SI joint injections, SI joint fusion (last resort)

Vertebral Body Osteomyelitis

- Vertebral body bacterial infection, which eats away at the bone and advances into the surrounding tissues, including spinal canal/cord

- Usually in the setting of IVDA, diabetes, immunocompromised status

- Usually staph aureus + lumbar spine

- Tuberculosis osteomyelitis occurs in at the thoracolumbar junction (Pott disease)

- Patient has signs and symptoms of infection + back pain; may develop neurologic deficits

- Workup: xrays, MRI with contrast (bright on T2), CBC, ESR, CRP, bone biopsy culture

- Treatment: ID consult, IV → oral antibiotics, surgery if stabilization or decompression required

Herniated Disc

- Squeezing of the intervertebral disc by compressive forces and/or annular tearing that causes the nucleus pulposus to shoot out posteriorly into the spinal canal
    - Usually due to heavy lifting, improper technique

- It can shoot out in different directions and with differing severities

- This herniation can cause inflammatory prostaglandins to be released, which is why epidural steroid injections (which decrease inflammation) can be effective for herniated discs causing radiculopathy

- Patient can complain of pain and/or weakness in a radicular (nerve root) distribution

    O   Usually L4-S1 or C5-C6 disc

Herniated Disc

- Workup: MRI

- **Bulging disc** = disc (nucleus + annulus) puffs out a little bit beyond the VB

- **Prolapsed disc** = nucleus leaks into the annulus

- **Extruded disc** = nucleus leaks all the way through the annulus to reach the PLL

- **Sequestered disc** = some nucleus material is separated off (sequestered) and hanging out by itself somewhere within the spinal canal

- In lumbar spine…

  - Central/paracentral disc herniation will involve the descending nerve root at that level

  - Posterolateral disc herniation will involve the descending nerve root at that level

  - Lateral disc herniation will involve the exiting nerve root at that level

  - E.g. L3-L4 central or posterolateral herniation will cause an L4 radiculopathy, whereas an L3-L4 lateral disc herniation will cause an L3 radiculopathy

Herniated Disc

- **Treatment**

  - Relative rest, PT with traction and directional preference assessment (McKenzie), acetaminophen, NSAIDs, neuropathic pain medications (gabapentin, pregabalin, amitriptyline), interlaminar or transforaminal epidural steroid injections (ESI/TFESI), surgical decompression (laminectomy)

Discogenic Pain

- Annulus fibrosus tearing, leading to midline back pain, typically worse with flexion, as this pulls on the torn annulus fibers and activates pain receptors in the process

  - Can be worse with sitting, extension, twisting

  - Typically due to VB endplate fractures which cause annulus tears

    - Note you can have leakage of the nucleus pulposus into the VB defect, and this is called a Schmorl node

- Tears can occur radially and be graded by how far they progress through the disc, from no annulus disruption to complete annulus disruption (Grade 0-3)

- **Workup:** MRI (may show high intensity zone [HIZ] within the annulus on T2 images), discogram

- **Treatment:** relative rest, PT, pain medications

Myelopathy

- Injury to the spinal cord from a huge variety of causes
  - Trauma, spondylosis, spinal stenosis, infection, cancer, MS, herniated disc
  - Note this may be acute or gradually progressive
- May cause weakness, UMN signs, spasticity, abnormal sensation, bowel/bladder/sexual dysfunction
- Patients often complain of progressive gait dysfunction in the context of the above symptoms
- +Babinski, +Hoffman, hyperreflexia, weakness, abnormal sensation
- **Workup:** MRI (cord signal change compared to noncompressed/healthy cord)
- **Treatment:** soft collar/bracing if mild and not debilitating (avoid high risk activities); IV steroids + emergent surgical decompression if acute presentation or severe and debilitating

Radiculopathy

- Radicular = "wraps around"
- **Radiculopathy** = weakness or abnormal sensation in a myotomal or dermatomal distribution, often due to herniated disc or spinal stenosis
  - Patients usually have back pain with this as well
  - +Spurling, cervical compression test, straight leg raise, slump sit, femoral nerve stretch test
- In the cervical spine, nerve roots exit above their VB level
- Below that, they exit just below their VB level
  - A C6,C7 disc herniation will cause a C7 radiculopathy
  - An L4,L5 lateral disc herniation will cause an L4 radiculopathy
  - An L4,L5 paracentral disc herniation will cause an L5 radiculopathy
- **Workup:** EMG/NCS, MRI
- **Treatment:** PT, epidural steroid injection directed at the nerve root in question, surgical decompression
- See EMG/NCS section for more detail

Back Strain/Sprain

- Essentially this is what most people have when they have "run of the mill" acute back pain
- This is a nonspecific muscle strain (pulled muscle) or ligament sprain in the back
- It is usually self-resolving
- Typically tender to palpation over involved muscle/ligament

- No neurologic deficits
- **Workup:** none
- **Treatment:** relative rest, ice, heat, PT, acetaminophen/NSAIDs

Myofascial Back Pain

- Painful tightness in the (usually) upper back and neck muscles with localized paresthesias due to tight fascia and muscles, often secondary to muscle weakness and poor posture
- These localized spots of tight, tender muscle and fascia are called trigger points
- Trigger points should be taut bands of tissue that, when pulled tight by the physician, reproduce the patient's pain and cause a localized, rippling, muscle twitching response
- Exacerbated by stress
- **Workup:** none
- **Treatment:** PT, counseling, heat/ice, trigger point injections

Chronic Back Pain

- Most people will experience back pain at some point in their lives
- The vast majority of back pains self-resolve within several weeks
- If you are out of work due to back pain, the longer you are out of work, the far less likely your chances of returning to work are
- Chronic back pain is often from a true structural back injury that just never improved, and over many months and years, various biochemical changes in the periphery and CNS have caused a centralization of pain perception, leading to a very difficult to treat chronic pain condition
- This often leads to unnecessary injections and surgeries

Interventional Spinal Procedures

- For in-depth discussion on board-relevant PM&R procedures, see Interventional PM&R section

The spine is a mystery to most doctors and a lot of physiatrists. But no longer to you!

Chapter 13: Pain Rehabilitation

Pain Rehabilitation

- Pain: unpleasant sensations usually secondary to acute tissue damage, but also can be due to chronic abnormalities of both neural and non-neural tissue
    - Dysesthesia: unpleasant sensation
    - Hyperesthesia: increased sensation
    - Hyperalgesia: increased pain from a normally painful stimulus
    - Allodynia: pain from a normally nonpainful stimulus (e.g. lightly touching the skin)
- Treating pain is an admirable goal in itself, but never forget that our ultimate goal is to improve function
    - It is a "win" if a patient's pain stays the same, but their function improves with our intervention
- Pain "sensation" occurs in different places
    - Damaged tissue: C fibers transmit pain impulses and send them to laminae 1, 2 in the dorsal horn
    - Spinal cord: dorsal horn accepts the stimulus, sends it up toward the thalamus and rest of brain
    - Brain: perception of painful sensation occurs in higher cognitive levels
- Pain can be **modulated** by doctors and the patient's body at any of these levels!

Pain Fibers

- Large, myelinated **Aβ fibers** transmit light touch and pressure impulses quickly to laminae 3-5 in the dorsal horn
- Small, unmyelinated **C fibers** transmit slow pain impulses to laminae 1,2 in the dorsal horn
- Both Aβ and C fibers synapse onto Wide Dynamic Range Neurons in the dorsal horn, which is why the **Gate Control Theory** of pain makes sense
    - Light touch, or essentially "rubbing a boo-boo" after it occurs, stimulates Aβ fibers, and when they synapse in the dorsal horn onto WDRNs, **this sends inhibitory signals to the C fiber synapses**, thus closing the gate on C fiber pain signal transmission
    - This is why you feel better when you scrape your knee and rub it lightly with your hand
    - This is why and how TENS units work!

Acute and Chronic Pain

- **Acute pain** occurs from damaged neural or non-neural tissue, with pain transmission along C fibers

- - Treatment is aimed at removing the insulting agent, controlling the pain perception, and breaking the cycle of acute pain as early as possible in order to **prevent the pain from becoming chronic**
- **Chronic pain** occurs from central biochemical changes that develop after weeks-months-years of uncontrolled acute pain, and is exacerbated by various psychosocial factors in a patient's life
  - Chronic pain is more difficult to treat, and often the goal becomes how to live with pain, rather than how to completely remove the pain
  - Chronic pain is far more resistant to typical treatment approaches (medications and procedures)

Pain Treatment

- Pain is treated with physical and occupational therapy, counseling, pain psychology, psychiatry, a wide array of pharmacologic approaches (see Pharmacology section), and interventional procedural approaches
- Do not forget the impact of psychological counseling and pain psychological approaches in terms of altering a patient's perception of chronic pain and how they allow it to affect their lives
  - Pain psychology is an important component of every chronic pain treatment program

Pain Syndromes and Treatments

- Note that throughout this series we have covered numerous painful conditions of the MSK and nervous systems that will not be re-discussed here; as a result this lecture is of course not an exhaustive list
- We will discuss a few pain syndromes that did not have a fair spotlight in earlier sections

Complex Regional Pain Syndrome (CRPS)

- AKA reflex sympathetic dystrophy (RSD), shoulder-hand syndrome
- Essentially this is sympathetically mediated pain due to an unknown etiology that results in an area of the body having increased neuropathic pain, hypersensitivity, and allodynia, all in conjunction with detectable skin and vasomotor changes over the affected area on the body
  - It typically occurs after trauma to an area of the body without nerve injury
- **CRPS Type 1** = the above symptoms **without** a known peripheral nerve injury
- **CRPS Type 2** = the above symptoms **within a known peripheral nerve distribution**
  - "Causalgia"

Complex Regional Pain Syndrome (CRPS)

- **CRPS has 3 stages**
  - **Stage 1: ACUTE**

- ■ Increased pain (burning/shooting), sweating (hyperhidrosis), swelling/edema, allodynia, vasomotor changes, hyperalgesia, increased hair growth
- ■ 3-6 months
- ○ Stage 2: DYSTROPHIC
  - ■ Continued pain, skin and nail atrophy, muscle atrophy
  - ■ 3-6 months
- ○ Stage 3: ATROPHIC
  - ■ Decreased pain, cool and shiny skin, skin and nail atrophy, muscle atrophy, hairlessness, lack of sweating, no edema, osteopenia, contractures
- ● Workup: xrays may show osteopenia; triple phase bone scan shows increased uptake in the 3rd phase; **stellate ganglion block is the gold standard diagnostic test**

Complex Regional Pain Syndrome (CRPS)

- ● **Treatment**
  - ○ MAINTAIN ROM to prevent contracture, learned disuse, and disuse atrophy
  - ○ TREAT EARLY to help "nip it in the bud" before it progresses out of control
  - ○ Prednisone 1 mg/kg PO DAILY spread throughout the day x2 weeks
  - ○ NSAIDs, gabapentin, pregabalin, carbamazepine, propranolol, nifedipine, topical lidocaine/diclofenac/capsaicin
  - ○ Desensitization in PT/OT
  - ○ TENS unit
  - ○ **Stellate ganglion block**, anesthetic/steroid injection, spinal cord stimulator

Headaches (Tension, Migraine, Cluster)

- ● **Tension Headaches**
  - ○ Most common headache; band-like throbbing pain around the head and temples
  - ○ Treat with hydration, rest, ice, acetaminophen, NSAIDs, myofascial trigger point injections, periscapular and cervical/upper back stretching and strengthening

- ● **Migraine Headaches**
  - ○ Typically unilateral, retro-orbital, pulsing headache that "seizes the moment" and is quite disabling when it occurs
  - ○ Common migraine occurs without an aura
  - ○ Classic migraine occurs with an aura off visual/auditory/neurologic dysfunction
  - ○ Occurs with photophobia and phonophobia (patient prefers a quiet, dark room)
  - ○ Etiology unknown; may be related to blood flow changes in the brain
  - ○ **ABORT** with triptan, acetaminophen, NSAIDs

- o **PREVENT** with propranolol, carbamazepine, valproate, gabapentin, pregabalin, TCAs, magnesium, botulinum toxin injections (migraine protocol chemodenervates a series of muscles in the upper face and head/neck)

Headaches (Tension, Migraine, Cluster)

- **Cluster Headaches**
    - o Severe, unilateral pain around one eye with conjunctival injection and tearing
    - o Headaches occur in clusters during the day/week/month/year
    - o **ABORT** with 100% oxygen
    - o **PREVENT** with anticonvulsants as with migraines (other medications are useful as well)
    - o Typically refer to neurologist for specialized headache management

Pelvic Pain

- Pelvic pain can be difficult to diagnose and treat, as its etiologies often don't fall square within the wheelhouse of a PM&R physician

- Pain in the pelvic region can be from a number of gynecologic diseases (ovary pathology, endometriosis, menstrual disorders, IBS, **interstitial cystitis** - inflamed bladder wall, diagnosed on cystoscopy with K^+ sensitivity test, treated with PT, counseling, diet changes, TCAs, cystoscopic procedures, surgery)

- Pelvic and groin pain can also be due to neuropathic etiology following surgery/procedure in the abdomen or pelvis, trauma, or idiopathic etiology
    - o Nerve blocks can improve or cure neuropathic pelvic pain
    - o **Genitofemoral, ilioinguinal, iliohypogastric** nerve blocks

Pain rehab is a short chapter. We cover a lot of pain pathologies in other chapters, so please think of this chapter as a "mopping up" of topics we had not covered yet prior to this chapter. And of course there's more. There's always more!

Chapter 14: Rheumatology

Rheumatology

- Joint and other organ system pathology due to a disorder of the immune system

- Rheumatologists specialize in treating these diseases medically

- Often the initial presentation is to a physiatrist

- Thus, it's important for us to have a good understanding of these diseases so that they can be diagnosed and treated in a timely fashion, as they often have disabling sequelae

- We'll talk about the most common high-yield rheumatologic diseases for the physiatrist to know

Rheumatoid Arthritis (RA)

- Autoimmune disorder causing symmetric systemic disease, including pathology in multiple joints

- Joints are destroyed by an inflammatory process (commonly knees, MCPs, PIPs, MTPs, C1-C2), caused by **pannus activity** (granulation tissue containing inflammatory cells)
  - The pannus destroys the joint cartilage, narrowing the joint space, leading to deformities

- Patient experiences morning stiffness lasting > 1 hour (improved with exercise), fatigue, fever, all usually gradually progressive over time (months)

Rheumatoid Arthritis

- RA diagnosis criteria change over time

- It is really not vital for the physiatrist to know the criteria cold

- Just know that in general patients have at least several weeks of joint pain ideally with positive RF/CCP and elevated ESR/CRP

- Labs: RF, anti-CCP antibodies, increased ESR/CRP

- Joint aspiration: cloudy, increased neutrophils (75%), < 100k WBC count
  - Septic arthritis has >100k WBCs, >75% neutrophils
  - Normal synovial fluid WBC count is nearly zero

Treatment of RA

- DMARD, DMARD, DMARD; doesn't matter how mild the disease is

- DMARDs are disease-modifying antirheumatic drugs that include methotrexate, hydroxychloroquine, sulfasalazine, infliximab, etanercept, adalimumab

- PT, OT for strength and ROM are vital

- NSAIDs help to decrease pain and inflammation

- Corticosteroids can be taken daily for chronic suppression in more severe disease

- Acutely inflamed joints: use isometric exercises

- Total joint replacements sometimes are needed

Sequelae of RA

- If not treated properly, RA leads to disability and disfigurement

- C1-C2 subluxation (atlantoaxial) can occur anteriorly
  - On flex-ex films there is a large gap between C1-C2 (>3mm)
  - May require fusion to prevent/treat cervical myelopathy

- **Radial** deviation of the wrist; **ulnar** deviation of the fingers
  - Treat with deviation-correcting orthoses

- Tenosynovitis of various tendons in wrist and ankle

- In general, ligaments can become disrupted and rupture
  - Ulnar collateral ligament rupture → floating ulnar head (piano key sign)

Sequelae of RA

- Swan neck deformity: DIP flexion, PIP extension, MCP flexion
  - Due to MCP/PIP synovitis
  - Treat with swan neck ring splint

- Boutonniere deformity: DIP extension, PIP flexion, MCP extension
  - Due to rupture of the PIP extensor hood which keeps the finger extensor lateral bands in place; thus, now the lateral bands sublux downward and essentially become flexors of the PIP while at the same time extending the DIPs like they normally would
  - The PIP pokes up through the two subluxed lateral bands like a poking a button through a buttonhole, hence the name
  - Treat with boutonniere ring splint

- Hallux valgus: great toe deviates laterally

- Hammer toes and claw toes can develop as well

- Finally, most major joints in the body can become inflamed and arthritic

- Multiple organ systems can become damaged, including pericarditis

Lupus (Systemic Lupus Erythematosus - SLE)

- Autoimmune disorder causing systemic inflammation

- Patients exhibit fatigue, nonerosive polyarthritis (unlike RA), malar rash, ANA+ (sensitive), anti-double-stranded DNA+ (specific), anti-Smith+ (specific), pericarditis, psychosis, renal dysfunction

- **Workup:** xrays of involved joints, labs as above including renal panel
- **Treatment:** immunosuppressants (azathioprine, mycophenolate mofetil, methotrexate), prednisone, NSAIDs, PT/OT

Gout

- Acute deposition of monosodium urate crystals into a joint, usually the great toe, causing acute synovitis which hurts a great deal
- Usually occurs to males who drink alcohol and eat red meat, or who take thiazides
- Fluid analysis reveals crystals with negative birefringence pattern
- Labs may show elevated uric acid, but we don't generally follow this
- Chronic tophi can develop (chronic uric acid deposition) which deform the joint
- **Treatment for acute attacks**
  - Indomethacin (first choice), colchicine, corticosteroids
- **Chronic prevention**
  - Allopurinol, febuxostat, probenecid

Pseudogout

- Also called chondrocalcinosis
- Due to acute calcium pyrophosphate crystal deposition, usually in the knee
- Can be seen idiopathically, or in metabolic disease such as thyroid disorders
- Synovial fluid analysis: envelope-shaped crystals with positive birefringence pattern
- Labs: normal uric acid
- **Treatment**
  - Indomethacin, colchicine, corticosteroids
  - Usually self-limiting

Septic Arthritis

- Fever/chills, joint pain/swelling/erythema, elevated WBC due to joint infection
  - Staph aureus in children; Neisseria gonorrhea in adults
- Workup: CBC, CMP, blood cultures, joint aspiration, xrays
  - Synovial fluid analysis will show >>>WBC (>100k) with overwhelming neutrophil predominance
- **Pott Disease**
  - Thoracolumbar junction vertebral body TB infection
- **Lyme Disease**
  - Joint infection with borrelia burgdorferi from a tick

- ○ Migratory polyarthritis involving the knee
- ○ Bullseye rash
- ○ **Treatment:** doxycycline

Polymyalgia Rheumatica (PMR)

- Proximal shoulder weakness and pain with fever
- **Workup:** ESR, CRP
- **Treatment:** prednisone, PT
- Maintain suspicion for temporal arteritis in these patients

Temporal Arteritis

- Inflammation of the temporal arteries, resulting in headache, jaw claudication, and potential blindness
- **Workup:** ESR (very high), CRP, temporal artery biopsy
- Blindness can result if not **treated with high-dose IV steroids ASAP**

Sjogren Syndrome

- Inflammation of ocular and oral glands, causing dry eyes and mouth, potentially joint pain
- **Workup:** ANA+, RF+
- **Treatment:** hydroxychloroquine, methotrexate

Raynaud Phenomenon

- This is a component of many rheumatologic diseases (Raynaud Disease is the phenomenon just by itself without other pathology) that involves vasospasm of the hand and feet blood vessels, usually due to cold temperature
- This can actually lead to necrosis of the fingers if severe
- **Treatment:** nifedipine, avoid offending causes (cold temperatures)

Scleroderma

- Systemic disease involving thickening/hardening of epithelial surfaces
- Involves skin thickening and arthritis
- Labs: ANA+
- **CREST** syndrome is a variety of scleroderma consisting of nephrocalcinosis, Raynaud phenomenon, esophageal dysmotility, sclerodactyly, telangiectasias
  - ○ CREST syndrome is ANA+, anti-centromere antibody+

Hemophilia

- Deficiency of clotting factor 8 (or 9 - Christmas Disease) that can lead to hemarthrosis, especially in the knee

- Acutely, may not want to drain the knee, as the blood tamponades further blood from entering

- Blood in the joint causes local inflammation, leading to erosive arthropathy

- **Treatment:** rest, PT, give them factor 8 or 9

Sickle Cell Arthropathy

- Abnormal RBC configuration leads to acute occlusion of the blood supply to bones and joints, leading to severe bone and joint pain

- Dactylitis very common

- Hip joint AVN very common

Seronegative Spondyloarthropathies (SEA)

- Arthritis involving the spine and multiple other sites/organs, without laboratory abnormalities (seronegative)

- HLA-B27+ (note that pauciarticular JRA is also HLA-B27+)

- Ankylosing spondylitis (AS), psoriatic arthritis, reactive arthritis, enteropathic arthritis (arthritis of IBD)

- **Ankylosing spondylitis**
  - Axial low back pain and stiffness typically in a young male
  - Ankylosis (fusion) can occur along the entire spine
  - +Schober test (<5cm excursion)
  - Xrays: **bilateral sacroiliitis,** bamboo spine (VB fusion and spinal ligament ossification)
  - **Treatment:** NSAIDs, steroids, DMARDs, firm mattress, sleep prone, PT for ROM and aerobics

Seronegative Spondyloarthropathies (SEA)

- **Psoriatic arthritis**
  - Arthritis associated with psoriasis (silvery scales on the skin)
  - Spine stiffness; multiple joint arthritis with "sausage fingers", DIP pencil-in-cup appearance (due to bone erosion around the joint); enthesopathy
  - **Treatment:** PT, ROM, NSAIDs, DMARDs, UV light for the skin

- **Reactive arthritis**
  - "Can't see, can't pee, can't climb a tree" → uveitis, urethritis, arthritis

- Occurs as a reaction after chlamydia/campylobacter/salmonella/other GI infection
- Asymmetric arthritis affecting especially the feet and ankles (can't climb a tree if you can't use your feet); enthesitis
- Xrays: plantar fascia and Achilles tendon insertion erosion
- **Treatment:** antibiotics, NSAIDs, PT

- **Enteropathic arthritis (arthritis of IBD)**
  - Arthritis due to IBD, especially in the knees
  - Treat the IBD and you will treat the arthritis (sulfasalazine, steroids)

Fibromyalgia

- Pain and tenderness to palpation over the entire body, classically at tender points along the posterior paramidline region, over past several months/years, typically in female patients

- Patients often have comorbid fatigue, anxiety, depression, lifestyle stressors

- Workup: none necessary

- Treatment: duloxetine, pregabalin, milnacipran, TCAs, PT, OT, **aquatherapy aerobics,** lifestyle modifications (sleep, home life, stressors, etc.), psychiatric management (SSRIs, counseling, pain psychology)

You're ready to be a rheumatologist! Or at least an expert in rheumatic physiatry. Wait, that sounds like a disease... How about you name it when you launch the subspecialty?

Chapter 15: EMG/NCS Overview

EMG/NCS

- **EMG** = electromyography
  - We stick needles into muscles, listen, then listen more as the muscle voluntarily contracts
- **NCS** = nerve conduction studies
  - We shock nerves and record further down the nerves to see how big the signal is, and how long it takes to get there
- Together they are called electrodiagnostic studies (EDX)
- Depending on what we see on EMG and NCS, we can diagnose what's going on with the patient
  - E.g. Why are they weak? Why are they numb?
- EMG/NCS only tests the peripheral nervous system
  - It tells us nothing about what's going on in the spinal cord or brain (i.e. CNS)

When to Order EDX

- Ordering EDX can be useful if the patient is weak in a particular muscle or group of muscles, or if they report numbness/tingling/altered sensation in one or more areas on their body
- Again, if the patient is weak or numb from a spinal cord injury alone, the EMG/NCS will essentially tell us nothing

Peripheral Nervous System

- Consists of sensory neurons and motor neurons
- **Sensory neurons**
  - Body (soma) is located in the dorsal root ganglion (DRG) adjacent to the spinal cord
  - These are called bipolar neurons because they have one projection that extends into the dorsal horn of the spinal cord to synapse there
  - **Dorsal column pathway (touch, pressure)**
    - DRG neuron will pass through the dorsal horn, then extend upward through the dorsal columns of the spinal cord (cuneate fasciculus and gracile fasciculus), synapse onto 2nd order neurons in the cuneate and gracile nuclei of the medulla, then decussate, continue to rise as the medial lemniscus, then synapse onto thalamus cells, which extend up into the parietal sensory cortex
  - **Spinothalamic pathway (pain, temperature)**
    - DRG neuron will rise a couple levels, then synapse onto the dorsal horn's 2nd order substantia gelatinosa cells, which will then decussate

and then rise as the spinothalamic tract until they synapse onto thalamus cells, which then project into the parietal sensory cortex

Peripheral Nervous System

- **Motor neurons**
  - AKA alpha motor neurons
  - Control of alpha motor neurons starts in the frontal lobe motor planning regions, which then send motor programs to the primary motor cortex, whose axons fire and transmit action potentials down the corticospinal tract, where they decussate in the medulla and synapse onto the anterior horns of the spinal cord
    - Interruption of this corticospinal tract pathway leads to loss of its descending inhibition upon alpha motor neurons; thus, muscles become hyperactive and **spasticity** results
  - Alpha motor neuron cell bodies start in the anterior horn of the spinal cord, and their axons project out all the way onto individual muscle cells, where they transmit their signal through the neuromuscular junction (NMJ) to cause the muscle cell to depolarize and release calcium from the sarcoplasmic reticulum, which causes myosin to bind to actin, causing the sarcomere to shorten

Peripheral Nervous System

- **Motor neurons**
  - One axon innervates many different muscle cells
  - An alpha motor neuron and all the muscle cells it innervates is called a **motor unit**
  - Different motor units have different **innervation ratios**
    - IR = #muscle fibers per alpha motor neuron
    - Huge, powerful muscles have huge innervation ratios
    - Small, fine motor muscles have small innervation ratios

Peripheral Nervous System

- **Myelin**
  - Schwann cells produce myelin, which wraps around axons and insulates them, protecting them and increasing their conduction velocity
  - When neurons lose myelin, they conduct action potentials more slowly

Nerve Anatomy

- **Endoneurium**
  - The connective tissue surrounding each individual axon and its myelin sheath
- **Perineurium**
  - The connective tissue connecting axons together into bundles (called nerve fascicles)

- **Epineurium**
    - The connective tissue connecting fascicles together
- On ultrasound, short axis view of a nerve, the nerve looks like a honeycomb because of these nerve fascicles
- When you sever a nerve (transection), you cut completely through the epineurium

Peripheral Nervous System

- **Neuromuscular junction (NMJ)**
    - The NMJ is how a neuron transmits its electrical action potential (AP) into the muscle cell
    - Ca^{2+} channels at the terminal part of the axon (near the NMJ) respond to the AP by letting Ca^{2+} into the axon
    - This Ca^{2+} causes synaptic vesicles (SNAP-25, syntaxin, synaptobrevin) to release their neurotransmitter contents (acetylcholine - ACh) into the synaptic cleft
    - ACh binds to ACh receptors on the muscle cell membrane, which then cause an electrical transmission through the muscle cell's T-tubule system, reaching the sarcoplasmic reticulum eventually, which then releases Ca^{2+} into the muscle cell, causing myosin to bind to actin and shorten the sarcomere
        - Thus, when lots of sarcomeres contract in unison, the entire muscle itself contracts
    - Botulinum toxin works by inhibiting the synaptic vesicles from releasing ACh into the synaptic cleft; thus, there's no way the muscle can ultimately receive a signal to contract, and the muscle becomes paralyzed

Peripheral Nervous System

- **ACh release**
    - ACh is released spontaneously at regular intervals, which cause miniature depolarizations (MEPPs) of the postsynaptic endplate (not enough to cause an action potential)
    - They are released as packets of ACh, called quanta
    - Action potentials of the presynaptic neuron cause a lot of quanta to be released into the synaptic cleft, generating EPPs
        - The EPP is usually much higher than required to generate an action potential

Action Potential

- The axonal membrane exists at a resting negative charge (-70 mV)
- The Na^+/ K^+ ATPase is the enzyme that exports 3 Na^+ for 2 K^+
- When an action potential travels along an axon, it opens up voltage-gated Na^+ channels
    - Thus, Na^+ rushes in and K^+ rushes out
    - Other channels (e.g. ion leak channels) help to re-establish equilibrium

- Myelin insulates this ion flow by shielding the membrane, thus forcing the action potential to jump from node of Ranvier to node of Ranvier (node = a gap in the myelin sheath)
  - This makes conduction fast!

Nerve Conduction Studies (NCS)

- These are usually Part 1 of the "EMG" test, with EMG needling being Part 2
- NCS involve applying current to sensory and motor nerves to measure how large and how fast the response is over the area of skin we choose to record
  - Shocking them and seeing if they look normal or abnormal
- This is done using a stimulating electrode, recording electrode, reference electrode, and ground electrode
  - Studies done on sensory nerves allow us to record a sensory nerve action potential = SNAP
  - Studies done on motor nerves allow us to record a compound muscle action potential = CMAP

Stimulating Electrode

- Typically a two-pronged device (like a tuning fork)
  - One of the prongs is the cathode (negatively charged)
  - One of the prongs is the anode (positively charged)
- When you want to stimulate a nerve, place the cathode over the spot you want to stimulate, with the anode "behind it"
  - I.e. the cathode is closer to the recording area of skin than the anode is
- The negatively charged cathode will attract + ions toward it, which will cause a LOT of Na^+ ions to accumulate outside the axon membrane, right where the cathode is above the skin
- This huge accumulation of Na^+ ions will eventually cause the voltage-gated Na^+ channels to open, thus initiating an action potential right there
  - It technically travels in both directions

Recording Electrode (G1)

- This can be a metal ring (useful for fingers), a bar, or tiny discs that you tape onto the skin to record
  - Also called the active electrode; it is usually marked black
- These record the action potential once you shock the nerve from a distance and the action potential travels all the way to the area of skin it innervates
  - Sensory nerve action potential (**SNAP**)
- It also records the action potential after it has traveled all the way down a motor nerve, transmitted through the NMJ, and caused muscle fiber depolarization

- Compound motor action potential (**CMAP**)
- Compound because although it is only one nerve, when you record it you are actually recording all the many muscle fibers that that nerve has caused to depolarize and contract
- Amplitude of the CMAP is a key prognostic factor, as it tells you how big the portion of healthy axons remaining is

Reference Electrode (G2)

- This is the same thing as the active electrode, only you place it over a neutral area like tendon or bone
  - Usually around 4 cm away from the active electrode; it is usually marked red
- Its purpose is to listen to all the electrical noise in the room and on the skin, and cancel out all the noise
- The idea is that the active electrode is *also* picking up these noise signals in addition to the action potential it is *intended to* pick up
- Because both electrodes can hear the noise, you can cancel out the noise
  - Like cancelling out the same thing both sides of an equation
  - Important in places like ICUs where there's a lot of machines that cause electrical noise
- A common interference frequency is 60 Hz interference, which shows up on your screen as a slow, steady wave

Ground Electrode

- Its purpose is to provide a safe pathway by which to dissipate current from the patient's body
- It is usually marked green
- It is usually placed between the stimulator and active electrode

The Signal Waveform

- The action potential, when recorded from the skin, shows up as a wave
  - Looks like a roller coaster
- We essentially look at how high the wave goes (amplitude), and how fast it arrived at the recording electrode (conduction velocity and latency)
- Let's draw out the action potential signal and learn what it means when we talk about the potential's amplitude, duration, onset latency, peak latency, conduction velocity, temporal dispersion

Orthodromic vs. Antidromic Recording

- Motor NCS are typically recorded orthodromically

- O The nerve is shocked and the AP travels down the axon just like it does in everyday life
- Sensory NCS are typically recorded antidromically
  - O The nerve is shocked proximal on the limb, and recording takes place distally
  - O This is weird, yes, but it gives us a better, louder signal from the nerve

Temperature Effects on the Action Potential

- Upper limbs should be kept at 32° C
- Lower limbs should be kept at 30° C
- If the limb is too cold, the amplitude will increase, CV will be slow with prolonged latency, and duration will increase
  - O Channels stay open longer, causing a beefier amplitude and longer time of depolarizing

Filters

- **High-frequency filter**
  - O Filters out noise above a certain frequency (Hz)
  - O Anything above its limit will be excluded from the final waveform display
  - O Also called a "low pass filter" because anything under it will be displayed
- **Low-frequency filter**
  - O Filters out noise below a certain frequency (Hz)
  - O Anything below its limit will be excluded from the final waveform display
  - O Also called a "high pass filter" because anything over it will be displayed
- Sensory NCS: typical filter settings are 20-2000 Hz
- Motor NCS: typical filter settings are 10-10,000 Hz

Adjusting the Filters

- If you lower the high frequency filter or raise the low frequency filter, you are essentially squishing the action potential down
  - O The amplitude is decreased
- Lowering the high frequency filter will also prolong the onset and peak latencies
  - O "I'm **late** because I was **high**"
- Raising the low frequency filter will also shorten the peak latency
  - O "I **peaked early** at a **low** point in my life"
  - O "**amp-low**-tude"

Age Effects on the Action Potential

- Normal upper extremity CV is at least 50 m/s

- Normal lower extremity CV is at least 40 m/s
- Once you reach age 50, your CV will decrease ~2 m/s per decade and this is normal

Using Too Much Current

- Normal range of current you will apply with your stimulator is 1-100 milliAmps with the duration of the shock lasting 0.1-1.0 ms
- Going well over this amount (often you will need much less than 100 milliAmps) is known as supramaximal stimulation and can cause volume conduction
- Supramaximal stimulation is a good practice to be sure that your waveform doesn't change in amplitude (i.e. you've reached maximum depolarization of all the nerve fibers), but if you continue to go higher and higher, you can cause volume conduction
- **Volume conduction** is the idea that applying too much current will cause the current to diffuse along tissues other than nerve, and your recording electrode will pick this up and alter the waveform
    - May see a falsely short latency or falsely fast conduction velocity

Skin Factors

- The patient having moisturizer or lotion on their skin will make NCS difficult
- Leads don't stick, pens don't write well

Motor NCS

- The motor NCS usually entails recording from the muscle belly and shocking the nerve at a distal location, a proximal location, and a more proximal location, etc.
- Theoretically the amplitude will be pretty much the same height at each shock location if all the axons are intact (there is a small amount of decrease normally)
- We only record the distal latency value and ignore the other latencies from more proximal stimulations
- The conduction velocity should be normal from each stimulation point
- Shocking at different spots means we can detect if there is CV slowing across a segment, which may indicate focal demyelination

H-Reflex

- Stimulating the Ia sensory afferent nerves and recording over the muscle will cause the AP to travel up to the spinal cord, stimulate the spinal reflex arc, and travel back down the motor nerve to make the muscle contract
    - It is a true reflex
- Recording electrode is placed over soleus
- Reference electrode is placed over achilles tendon
- Stimulate in proximal direction from the popliteal fossa

- This response should have a symmetric latency from side to side, and should be in the range of normal for the patient's age group
- If prolonged latency, this indicates that there is damage *somewhere* along that entire reflex pathway
  - Thus, it is nonspecific
  - Frequently used to assess for S1 radiculopathy

F-Wave

- The F-wave (or F reflex) is produced when recording from a muscle and stimulating the nerve of that muscle at a distal location in a proximal stimulation direction
  - E.g. recording over FDI, antidromically stimulating ulnar nerve at wrist
- This will send an AP antidromically back up, all the way to the anterior horn, which will then cause depolarization of a random population of anterior horn cells, whose depolarization will then travel back down the axons of the motor nerve and will be recorded by our recording electrode over the muscle belly
- Thus, it is not actually a true reflex
- Can generally be obtained from any motor nerve
- Normal if you see an F-wave on 80% or more of your stimulations, and if they are all similar in terms of latency
- Also not very specific since you are evaluating a long motor pathway
  - **However, prolonged/absent F-Waves are the first sign of Guillain Barre syndrome**

A-Wave

- Also called the axon reflex (also not a true reflex)
- This is a very predictable, stable waveform that shows up somewhere between the F-Wave and the direct motor response when recording F-Waves from a muscle
- It is the same exact waveform with every stimulation
  - Same latency and amplitude
- If you see A-Waves, it usually means there has been reinnervation of the nerve to that muscle (i.e. prior nerve damage occurred at some point in the patient's life)

Electromyography (EMG)

- In EMG we advance needles into muscles and listen to the muscle's electrical activity, both at rest and with voluntary activation
  - The needle is essentially a fine, thin wire
- We typically use concentric or monopolar electrodes to do this
- **Concentric**

- ○ Has a small listening area
- ○ Reference electrode is attached to the needle
- **Monopolar**
  - ○ Has a very broad listening area
  - ○ Reference electrode is separate and needs to be attached to the skin surface
- With these needles we assess **insertional activity, resting activity, and recruitment**
- With recruitment, we are assessing the frequency of firing, the size, and the shape of motor unit action potentials (**MUAPs**)

Insertional Activity

- This refers to the sounds and visual patterns on the screen that emit from the electrode with each abrupt, sharp advancement further into the muscle
- When inserting through skin and subcutaneous tissue, the sound is generally muffled
- When reaching muscle, a crisp "TV static / record scratch" type of noise is abruptly heard with each moment of needle advancement
  - ○ These are electrical potentials you are creating by ripping through the muscle
- Insertional activity is either decreased (fibrosis), normal, or increased (active denervation)
- The level of insertional activity will immediately clue you in on what type of pathology the patient may have, if any

Resting Activity

- In a normal muscle at rest, you will hear either **total silence, MEPPs/seashell noise** (when you are near endplates which are painful for the patient), **EPPs** due to needle causing EPPs to be produced, or **abnormal spontaneous activity** (fibs and sharps).
- Fibrillations and positive sharp waves (fibs and sharps) occur as regular spikes with a regular popping sound
  - ○ If the spike peaks in the downward direction, it is a PSW
  - ○ Their regularity of firing tells you what they are
  - ○ **They indicate active denervation (axonal loss)** occurring in that muscle
  - ○ That denervation can be from a root-level injury, plexus injury, peripheral nerve injury, etc.
- Abnormal spontaneous activity (fibs and sharps) is graded as 0 to 4+
- 0 being normal and 4+ meaning the whole screen is filled with fibs and sharps
  - ○ Like a house that's on fire

Resting Activity

- **Fibs and sharps** (discussed; indicate active denervation of that muscle)

- **Fasciculations**
  - Involuntary potentials due to spontaneous muscle contractions
  - They look like normal MUAPs and fire irregularly
  - Seen in anterior horn cell disease (numerous) and normal patients

- **Myokymia**
  - Involuntary, abrupt, fairly regular "marching" potentials, tightly grouped together
  - Sound like soldiers marching
  - Seen in upper trunk radiation plexopathy

Resting Activity

- **Complex repetitive discharge (CRD)**
  - Involuntary, similar to myokymic discharges, except the whole discharge is much wider and very serrated like a saw (thus it is complex in appearance, and repetitive in firing)
  - Due to a motor unit becoming denervated, then reinnervated by another motor neuron, which then also becomes denervated
  - *Ephaptic transmission* is the process by which these muscle fibers all fire regularly together
  - Seen in chronic radiculopathy, anterior horn cell disease, normal patients

- **Myotonic discharge**
  - Involuntary potentials that are heard when you move the needle into an affected muscle fiber
  - The amplitude steadily decreases as the muscle fiber continues to fire
  - It sounds like a **divebomber**
  - Seen in anything with "myotonia" or similar in its name
    - Myotonic dystrophy, paramyotonia, myotonia congenita AND hyperkalemic periodic paralysis, acid maltase deficiency

Recruitment

- This refers to the patient voluntarily activating their alpha motor neurons with gradually increasing intensity
- The alpha motor neurons will "recruit" the muscle fibers that belong to them to contract
  - Motor units sequentially activate, with the smallest motor units being activated first
  - Huge motor units, which often contain Type II muscle fibers, are activated with maximal intensity, which will fill the screen with motor units (called a normal, maximal interference pattern)
- Normally, you start with one motor unit (MUAP) firing at a rate of 5 Hz

- If you increase your contraction intensity slightly, this motor unit will increase its firing rate to 10 Hz, AND you will now recruit a second motor unit which will start firing at 5 Hz
- You should be able to get 4 MUAPS on the screen, firing at 20/15/10/5 Hz

Decreased Recruitment

- Count how many times a single MUAP shows up on the screen and multiply by 5
  - This will tell you the Hz (ballpark estimate)
  - E.g. you see the same MUAP 4 times → it is firing at about 20 Hz
- **Decreased recruitment** occurs if there has been axonal damage, and now only *some* of the alpha motor neurons can actually activate muscle fibers
- With decreased recruitment, you see an *increased firing rate* of MUAPs
  - Imagine that so many axons have died, that there is only one axon left
  - In order to cause the muscle to contract with sufficient force, this axon is going to have to fire *so fast* in order to pick up the slack caused by the other dead axons' absence
  - Decreased recruitment kind of sounds like a machine gun
  - You may see firing rates of 30, 40, 50 Hz with only 1-2 MUAPs on the screen, *doing all the work*
- This is sometimes called a *neuropathic recruitment pattern*, because it indicates that there is some kind of neuropathy going on (rather than a muscle problem - myopathy)

Decreased Recruitment

- Axonal loss will show up as decreased recruitment as discussed
- The MUAPS will not only be more scarce, with each one firing faster than it normally should, but over time each one will also be large and long
  - Large amplitude, long duration (LDLA) MUAPs = neuropathic MUAPs
- They become large because axons that have not died will actually demonstrate **collateral sprouting** and take over muscle fibers that used to belong to dead axons
- These collateral sprouts are not uniformly myelinated at first, so due to variations in how consistently the APs are transmitted to all the neuron's muscle fibers, the MUAP will initially be **polyphasic** (crosses the baseline 5 or more times)
  - Polyphasic MUAPs are also called **reinnervation potentials**
- The large amplitude, long duration shape of the reinnervated MUAP occurs due to that neuron recruiting *a lot more* muscle fibers, enlarging the MUAP

Increased Recruitment

- Conversely, if the neurons are all intact, but the muscle is diseased, then in order to actually get a strong contraction out of the muscle, it's going to take recruiting all of the muscle fibers in order to actually get the muscle to contract
    - Each of the muscle fibers is so weak (due to disease), that literally all of them may have to contract at once in order for the muscle to actually do anything
- This means that with very small effort, we see the screen become flooded with many, many small, short MUAPs
    - Like using a thousand weak, little pinky fingers to collectively lift an anvil
- This is called **increased recruitment** and is typically due to myopathy
    - Thus, it is sometimes called a *myopathic recruitment pattern*
    - Small duration, small amplitude motor units (SDSA) = myopathic motor units

Demyelination vs. Axonal Loss

- **Demyelination**
    - A focal or diffuse removal of myelin around an axon
    - Due to focal compression (e.g. CTS), stretching, systemic disease (e.g. AIDP), etc.
    - Action potentials don't travel as fast in unmyelinated/demyelinated nerves
        - NCS: Prolonged latency, decreased CV, increased temporal dispersion
        - EMG: normal (no conduction block) vs. decreased recruitment (conduction block)

- **Axonal loss**
    - Degeneration of axons
    - Due to focal crush, transection, stretching, systemic disease, anterior horn cell disease, etc.
    - Very few healthy axons exist to summate into the CMAP
        - NCS: decreased amplitude (possibly decreased CV if fastest fibers are destroyed)
        - EMG: decreased recruitment
    - Axonal vs. Wallerian degeneration
        - Retrograde vs. anterograde processes
        - Wallerian degeneration is complete by 5 days (motor) or 10 days (sensory)

Conduction Block

- **Conduction block** is the failure of an action potential to propagate past a focal spot in the peripheral nervous system, while the ability to conduct action potentials beyond that particular spot is preserved

- It is essentially like driving up to a bridge only to find out that there is a huge gap in the middle of it
    - You can drive up to the bridge
    - You can drive onward if you just start on the other side of the bridge
    - **But you cannot cross the bridge = action potentials cannot cross = conduction block**
- This means that when we are trying to measure CMAPs (amplitude, CV, latency) we can't really do that if we are trying to stimulate the nerve proximal to the spot of conduction block
- The CMAP looks normal if we stimulate distal to the conduction block

Conduction Block

- **What is causing the conduction block?**
    - Focal area of demyelination that essentially short circuits the affected axons at that spot
    - This can mean TOTAL conduction block in which you see zero amplitude if trying to conduct proximally to the lesion and record at the distal muscle belly
    - It can also just mean PARTIAL conduction block in which only some of the amplitude is lost (e.g. only some of the axons are short-circuited) when trying to conduct our stimulus across the lesion
- **What causes the demyelination?**
    - Often focal compression (CTS, Saturday Night Palsy, any prolonged compression of any nerve)
    - Sometimes GBS can cause conduction block at what are typically *non-entrapment sites,* which can clue you in to the GBS diagnosis

Conduction Block

- **Important point to remember:**
    - When you try to stimulate a nerve proximally, and you see a low amplitude, you may be tempted to diagnose axonal loss due to the amplitude being low
    - Be sure to stimulate very distally to see if the amplitude is recorded as normal
    - If the amplitude is in fact normal distally, you have a conduction block somewhere along that nerve

Seddon Nerve Injury Classifications

- **Neurapraxia**
    - Focal pressure on a nerve, causing focal demyelination, leading to conduction block
    - Axons are intact, so if you stimulate distally, everything (CMAP) looks normal

- If you stimulate proximally, you see decreased amplitude, but if you wait a few weeks and then stimulate proximally again, everything looks normal due to remyelination

- **Axonotmesis**
  - Crush or stretch injury to nerve, leading to axon death with the epineurium still intact
  - Thus, even though axons have died, there is still intact epineurium which will serve as a guide path for the axons to regenerate along and ultimately find their target muscle fibers again
  - Immediately you see decreased amplitude proximally, normal CMAP distally
  - After a few weeks you see decreased amplitude proximally and distally with fibs and sharps on EMG and decreased recruitment
  - Weeks to months later you can see reinnervation potentials (polyphasic MUAPs)
  - Axons grow about 1 inch per month, so eventually the regenerated axons may return to their former muscle fibers which are now reinnervated by other motor neurons
  - The biggest motor neuron with the strongest NMJ connection will "win" control of the muscle fiber

Seddon Nerve Injury Classifications

- **Neurotmesis**
  - Completely severing (transecting) the nerve, all the way through the epineurium, due to trauma
  - Initially we see absent CMAP proximally, normal CMAP distally
  - Once Wallerian degeneration is complete after about 5 days (for motor fibers), we see absent CMAP **both** proximally and distally
  - This time if we wait a few weeks and stimulate again, we will still see absent CMAPs both proximally and distally
  - **Why?**
    - Because the epineurium is completely severed, so there is no way for those axons to ever grow back; they have no pathway to guide them (normally intact epineurium could serve as a guide path for regenerating axons)
  - In addition, on EMG, we will see fibs and sharps with absent recruitment
  - A neuroma can form as these axons attempt (poorly) to find their muscle fibers again while the axons are regenerating. This neuroma can be painful and cause paresthesias locally. It can be identified on MRI, ultrasound, and it can be resected or injected with lidocaine and steroid

Blink Reflex Study (NCS)

- The blink reflex study is used to detect lesions of the trigeminal nerve, facial nerve, and pons/medulla

- ○ Useful in strokes, MS, trauma
- Before we look at how we study it, we need to know the simple pathway that it is studying

Blink Reflex Study (NCS)

- Facial sensation is via the trigeminal nerve (V)
- Facial motor control is via the facial nerve (VII)
- V sensory input is conducted from the face all the way into the pons where the V nucleus is located (called Vm)
- This input is then conducted from the V nucleus directly to the ipsilateral VII nucleus (also in pons) which will reflexively cause a blink response via VII output to the orbicularis oculi muscle
  - ○ This quick, ipsilateral blink response is called the **R1 response** and we record it from the orbicularis oculi muscle ipsilaterally to the stimulation side
- At the same time that the Vm nucleus conducts its impulse to the ipsilateral VII nucleus for the above to take place, the Vm nucleus also conducts the impulse to the medulla, where...

Blink Reflex Study (NCS)

- ...where there sits another V nucleus called Vs
- Vs takes this impulse from Vm and sends it to bilateral VII nuclei, which causes a bilateral blink via the orbicularis oculi muscles
  - ○ These orbicularis oculi muscle contractions bilaterally are recorded as the ipsilateral and contralateral **R2 response**
- So that is a lot of verbal imagery
- Let's draw it out together to make sense of it

Blink Reflex Study (NCS)

- Sometimes you will be asked to interpret a blink reflex study
- Let's go through some common pathologies to get a hang of it

Blink Reflex Study (NCS)

- **Synkinesis**
  - ○ A complication of facial nerve regeneration
  - ○ Inaccurate, imprecise facial nerve reinnervation of target structures after the nerve has been damaged, leading to the nerve reinnervating muscles inappropriately, in such a fashion that you may end up doing 2 things at once when you only meant to do one of them
    - ■ E.g. blinking and moving your mouth at the same time

■ E.g. crying or salivating when moving facial muscles

EMG/NCS Overview Conclusion

- If you understand this lecture as well as the innervation pathways of most of the upper and lower extremity muscles, then the next section on EMG/NCS diseases will be a **breeze**

- Let's take a break now, and I'll see you in the next section

You know, pretty much all I would say is right above here. I'll give you a breather from the bad jokes. For now!

Chapter 16: Upper Extremity Peripheral Nervous System Diseases

Peripheral Nervous System Diseases

- Involve damage to motor and/or sensory nerves outside the brain and spinal cord

- Damage to motor and sensory nerves will show up as a certain pattern of injury on EMG/NCS, which is why these types of diseases are best evaluated with EMG/NCS (and imaging such as MRI, US)

- We will cover upper extremity neuropathies, lower extremity neuropathies, spinal pathologies, systemic neuropathies, and myopathies

- Knowing the EMG/NCS Overview section and peripheral nervous system/muscle innervations will make this section very simple and easy to follow

  o See lists on following slides; I will not insult your intelligence by reading these to you, but do take the time to memorize them via repetition (flash cards are great)

List of Upper Extremity Muscle Innervations
- **Muscle Innervations**
- C3, C4; spinal accessory nerve → trapezius, SCM
- C4, C5; dorsal scapular nerve (pre-plexus) → rhomboids
- C5, C6; upper trunk; suprascapular nerve → supraspinatus (then nerve passes through spinoglenoid notch) → infraspinatus
- C5, C6; upper trunk; lateral cord; musculocutaneous nerve → biceps brachii, brachialis
- C5, C6; upper trunk; posterior cord; axillary nerve → deltoid, teres minor
- C5, C6; upper trunk; posterior cord; radial nerve → BR
- C5, C6, C7; long thoracic nerve → serratus anterior
- C5, C6, C7, C8, T1; upper, middle, lower trunk; medial and lateral cord; medial and lateral pectoral nerves → Pec major
- C6, C7; upper and middle trunk; lateral cord; median nerve → PT, FCR
- C6, C7; upper and middle trunk; posterior cord; radial nerve → ECRL
- C6, C7, C8; upper, middle, lower trunk; posterior cord; radial nerve → triceps, anconeus
- C6, C7, C8; upper, middle, lower trunk, posterior cord; thoracodorsal nerve → latissimus dorsi
- C7, C8; middle and lower trunk; posterior cord; radial nerve; PIN → ECU, EIP, ED
- C7, C8; middle and lower trunk; medial and lateral cord; median nerve → FDS
- C7, C8, T1; middle and lower trunk; medial and lateral cord; median nerve; AIN → PQ, FPL
- C7, C8, T1; middle and lower trunk; medial cord; median nerve; AIN → FDP 2,3
- C7, C8, T1; middle and lower trunk; medial cord; ulnar nerve → FDP 4, 5
- C8, T1; lower trunk; medial cord; median nerve → APB, FPB, lumbricals 1,2, opponens pollicis
- C8, T1, lower trunk; medial cord; ulnar nerve → FCU, ADM, FDI, lumbricals 3,4, interossei (3 PADs and 4 DABs)
- **Cutaneous Innervations**
- C5, C6; upper trunk; lateral cord; musculocutaneous nerve; terminates as lateral antebrachial cutaneous nerve (LAC) → skin over lateral forearm

- C8, T1; lower trunk; medial cord; medial antebrachial cutaneous nerve (MAC) → skin over medial forearm

List of Lower Extremity Muscle Innervations

- **Muscle Innervations**
- L2, L3, L4; femoral nerve → quads, iliopsoas
- L2, L3, L4; obturator nerve → adductors; gracilis
- L4, L5; sciatic nerve; deep fibular nerve → tibialis anterior (TA), extensor digitorum longus (EDL)
- L4, L5, S1; sciatic nerve; deep fibular nerve → extensor hallucis longus (EHL), extensor digitorum brevis (EDB)
- L4, L5, S1; sciatic nerve (tibial division) → semimembranosus, semitendinosus, long head of biceps femoris
- L5, S1; sciatic nerve (fibular division) → short head of biceps femoris
- L4, L5, S1; superior gluteal nerve → gluteus medius, gluteus minimus, tensor fascia lata (TFL)
- L5, S1; sciatic nerve; superficial fibular nerve → fibularis longus, fibularis brevis
- L5, S1; sciatic nerve; tibial nerve → tibialis posterior (TP), flexor digitorum longus (FDL)
- L5, S1, S2; inferior gluteal nerve → gluteus maximus
- S1, S2; sciatic nerve; tibial nerve → gastrocnemius, soleus
- S1, S2; sciatic nerve; tibial nerve; medial plantar nerve → flexor hallucis brevis (FHB), abductor hallucis brevis (AHB)
- S1, S2; sciatic nerve; tibial nerve; lateral plantar nerve → abductor digiti quinti pedis (ADQP)
- **Cutaneous Innervations**
- L2, L3; lateral femoral cutaneous nerve → lateral thigh
- L2, L3, L4; femoral nerve; saphenous nerve → medial shin, medial calf
- L4, L5; sciatic nerve; tibial nerve; medial plantar nerve → medial plantar surface of foot
- S1, S2; sciatic nerve; tibial nerve; lateral plantar nerve → lateral plantar surface of foot

Upper Extremity Neuropathies

- Median neuropathy

- Anterior interosseous neuropathy

- Ulnar neuropathy

- Radial neuropathy

- Posterior interosseous neuropathy

- Axillary neuropathy

- Musculocutaneous neuropathy

- Suprascapular neuropathy

- Long thoracic neuropathy

- Brachial plexopathy

- *Note: almost all of these are amenable to in-office diagnostic ultrasound scan to evaluate if the nerve in question appears compressed, swollen, different from the other side, etc.*

Median Neuropathy

- Injury to the median nerve fibers (C6-T1 roots) at any site along the course of the nerve
- Injury is typically due to compression or trauma
- Proximal median neuropathy
  - AKA median neuropathy at the elbow
- Distal median neuropathy
  - AKA median neuropathy at the wrist (carpal tunnel syndrome)
- Let's discuss median neuropathy at the wrist (CTS) first

Median Neuropathy at the Wrist (CTS)

- Classically this is due to median nerve compression within the carpal tunnel of the wrist
- The carpal tunnel contains 10 structures within it
  - 4 FDS tendons, 4 FDP tendons, 1 FPL tendon, median nerve
- The carpal tunnel inlet is bordered by the scaphoid radially, then lunate and triquetrum on the floor, then ulnarly the pisiform bone
- Running over the top of the carpal tunnel is the transverse carpal ligament (AKA flexor retinaculum)
- Most of the time CTS is due to tight compression of the median nerve underneath this transverse carpal ligament

Median Neuropathy at the wrist (CTS)

- Pain at wrist/hand, weakness of hand (thumb abduction/opposition), numbness and tingling in first 3 ½ digits (median nerve distribution), worse at night; shaking their hands out at night may improve symptoms
- If they have symptoms in other digits, it is still probably median neuropathy at the wrist causing their symptoms
  - Sensation is subjective but EMG/NCS is objective
- Positive Tinel at wrist, Phalen, carpal compression test, +/- thenar atrophy
- **NCS**
  - Abnormal median SNAP to thumb, digit 2, digit 3
  - Abnormal median CMAP to APB
- **EMG**
  - Normal vs. decreased recruitment +/- fibs/sharps, polyphasicity

Median Neuropathy at the Wrist (CTS)

- Proximal median nerve EMG studies will be normal
  - PT, FCR, FDS
  - FPL, PQ, FDP (all anterior interosseous nerve)

- **Treatment**
  - If mild, carpal tunnel wrist splints at night; consider carpal tunnel injection
  - If moderate/severe, consider surgical release of flexor retinaculum

Median Neuropathy at the Elbow

- Similar presentation as CTS, except this is a compression of the median nerve at the elbow, typically by a tight pronator teres (PT) muscle, tight bicipital aponeurosis, or tight ligament of Struthers
  - Any of these can squeeze the median nerve and cause a compressive neuropathy

- Patient may have weakness of wrist flexion (FCR), PIP flexion (FDS), thumb flexion (FPL), DIP flexion of digits 1,2 (FDP 1,2), pronation (PQ)
  - In PT syndrome, usually the PT is spared because its innervation occurs more proximally

- **NCS**
  - Abnormal median SNAP and CMAP

- **EMG**
  - Decreased recruitment +/- fibs/sharps in every median muscle except PT (if PT syndrome)
  - Polyphasicity

Median Neuropathy at the Elbow

- If compression of median nerve takes place at ligament of Struthers or bicipital aponeurosis, then all median nerve muscles will be affected
- If compression takes place at PT, then all will be affected **except PT**
- **Treatment**
  - Rehab vs. US-guided nerve decompression (hydrodissection) vs. surgical release

Anterior Interosseous Neuropathy

- The AIN is actually a pure motor branch of the median nerve
- It branches off in the forearm to innervate the FPL, FDP 2,3, and PQ
  - Basically the "P" muscles
- Patient cannot make an "OK" sign or make a fist
- Injury is usually due to trauma or compression

- Thus, an AIN-opathy would have normal NCS and abnormal EMG to these muscles
- **NCS**
  - Normal median SNAPs and CMAP
- **EMG**
  - Abnormal activity (fibs/sharps), decreased recruitment in FPL, FDP 2,3, and PQ; polyphas
- **Treatment**
  - Rehab vs. US-guided decompression vs. surgery to remove compression source

Ulnar Neuropathy

- The ulnar nerve (C8, T1; lower trunk; medial cord; ulnar nerve) carries cutaneous innervation to the 4th and 5th digits (actually only 1/2 of the 4th digit), as well as motor control to the FCU, FDP 4,5, lumbricals 3,4, interossei (3 PADs and 4 DABs), ADM, FDI)
- Injury (compression or trauma) can occur both proximally and distally, just like with the median nerve
- **Proximal injury** occurs at the cubital tunnel (two heads of the FCU pinching the ulnar nerve) or Arcade of Struthers (fascia connecting brachialis to triceps)
- Sometimes a "tardy ulnar nerve palsy" occurs many months after a distal humerus fracture; altered biomechanics and osteophytes, etc., at the elbow can lead to the development of ulnar nerve compression/stretching
- **Distal injury** occurs at Guyon's Canal

Ulnar Neuropathy at the Wrist (Guyon's Canal)

- Compression of the ulnar nerve within Guyon's Canal
  - Roof = ligament (no need to know the name)
  - Floor = flexor retinaculum, hypothenar muscles
  - Medial border = pisiform
  - Lateral border = hook of the hamate
- The ulnar nerve can be compressed at different locations within Guyon's Canal (usually by bicyclists or ganglion cysts), causing different clinical pictures:
- **Type I** = motor and sensory
- **Type II** = motor
- **Type III** = sensory

Ulnar Neuropathy at the Wrist (Guyon's Canal)

- Patient complains of weakness in the hand (intrinsic hand muscle weakness), paresthesias in digits 4 and 5
- Positive Wartenberg and Froment signs

- Weakness in FDI, ADM, finger adduction and abduction, ulnar lumbricals
- NCS
  - Abnormal ulnar SNAPs to digits 4 and 5, abnormal CMAP to ADM, FDI
  - NORMAL dorsal ulnar cutaneous nerve (DUC) SNAP because the DUC branches off to innervate the skin PROXIMAL TO GUYON'S CANAL

- EMG
  - Abnormal activity (decreased recruitment, +/- fibs and sharps) to ulnar hand muscles (ADM, FDI, interossei, lumbricals 3 and 4); polyphasicity
  - Normal activity in proximal ulnar muscles (FCU, FDP 4, 5)

- Treatment
  - Rehab, discontinue offending activities, surgical release

Ulnar Neuropathy at the Elbow

- Similar symptoms of ulnar neuropathy at the wrist; may have vague elbow or forearm pain / tightness
  - Tight Arcade of Struthers, cubital tunnel syndrome,

- Positive Wartenberg and Froment signs AND weakness of wrist flexion, DIP flexion of digits 4, 5

- NCS
  - Abnormal ulnar SNAPs to digits 4 and 5, abnormal CMAP to ADM, FDI
  - Abnormal DUC, normal MAC SNAP

- EMG
  - Abnormal activity (decreased recruitment, +/- fibs and sharps) to ulnar hand muscles (ADM, FDI, interossei, lumbricals 3 and 4); polyphasicity
  - Abnormal activity in proximal ulnar muscles (FDP 4,5) (+/- FCU); polyphasicity

- Treatment
  - Rehab, discontinue offending activities, surgical release

Radial Neuropathy

- Injury to the radial nerve, usually due to compression or trauma, typically at the axilla (crutches), midshaft of the humerus (spiral groove), or proximal forearm

- Radial nerve innervates triceps, anconeus, brachioradialis, ECRL / ECRB
  - Sensory innervation to posterior arm, posterior forearm, thumb, snuffbox

- PIN is a branch of radial nerve that is pure motor and innervates other muscles

- Patient has wrist drop, finger drop, numbness / tingling in posterior forearm / thumb

- Compression can occur at various sites, leading to different EDX findings

- Patients typically have wrist drop, so rehab often involves ordering a wrist cockup splint to provide tenodesis (grip) action

Radial Neuropathy at the Elbow

- Weakness of wrist extensors and finger extensors with numbness and tingling in posterior forearm and thumb/snuffbox
  - ECRL/ERCB, EIP, ED, ECU
  - Elbow flexion may be weak with BR involvement
- Often due to compression between brachialis and brachioradialis where it sits
- **NCS**
  - Abnormal SNAP to thumb and snuffbox
  - Abnormal CMAP to EIP
- **EMG**
  - Abnormal activity in all radial muscles except triceps and anconeus
- **Treatment**
  - Rehab, remove offending agent, surgical release/transposition

Radial Neuropathy at the Spiral Groove

- Similar presentation as at the elbow, except often there is a history of midshaft humerus fracture or prolonged compression of something against the midshaft of the humerus (spiral groove) (Honeymooner's Palsy, Saturday Night Palsy)
- Elbow extension is normal (triceps, anconeus)
- **NCS**
  - Abnormal SNAP to thumb and snuffbox
  - Abnormal CMAP to EIP
- **EMG**
  - Abnormal activity in all radial muscles except triceps and anconeus
- **Treatment**
  - Rehab, remove offending agent, surgical release/transposition

Radial Neuropathy due to Improper Crutch Use

- Compression of crutches against the axillae causes a posterior cordopathy, which impairs all radial nerve innervation, period
- Elbow extension is weak and posterior arm sensation is impaired; otherwise same complaints as prior slides
- **NCS**
  - Abnormal SNAP to thumb and snuffbox
  - Abnormal CMAP to EIP

- **EMG**
  - Abnormal activity in all radial muscles INCLUDING triceps and anconeus
  - +/- abnormal activity in axillary-innervated muscles (posterior cord!)
- **Treatment**
  - Rehab, remove offending agent, surgical release/transposition

Superficial Radial Neuropathy

- The superficial radial nerve is what's left of the radial nerve after the PIN splits off in the proximal forearm
- It supplies sensation to posterior forearm, dorsal side of hand (thumb, snuffbox)
- Injury is due to compression/trauma (tight handcuffs, IV)
- Patient has numbness/tingling/burning pain in dorsal hand (thumb, snuffbox region)
- **NCS**
  - Abnormal SNAP to thumb and snuffbox
  - Normal CMAP to EIP
- **EMG**
  - Normal
- **Treatment**
  - Remove compression source, stop stabbing it with an IV, etc.

Posterior Interosseous Neuropathy (PIN)

- PIN is a pure motor branch of the radial nerve that branches off in the anterior elbow right between brachialis and BR, diving deep into the posterior compartment
- PIN is injured by compression (Arcade of Frohse), trauma (Monteggia fracture)
- Patient complains of aching proximal forearm pain with impaired finger extension (ED, EIP, EPL), wrist extension (ECU) with NORMAL SENSATION
- **NCS**
  - Normal SNAPs to radial, ulnar, median nerves
  - Abnormal CMAP to EIP
- **EMG**
  - Abnormal activity in all PIN muscles +/- supinator
  - ECRL, ECRB, BR, triceps, anconeus are all spared
- **Treatment**
  - Rehab, surgical decompression/release

Axillary Neuropathy

- Injury to the axillary nerve, usually due to trauma, stretching, compression, improper crutch use
- Axillary nerve innervates deltoid, teres minor, lateral arm skin (over deltoid)
- Wraps around through the quadrilateral space of the armpit underneath the GHJ
- Patient has shoulder abduction and external rotation weakness with impaired sensation over deltoid
- **NCS**
  - SNAP unavailable
  - Abnormal CMAP to deltoid
- **EMG**
  - Abnormal activity in deltoid, teres minor
- **Treatment**
  - Rehab, remove compression source, surgery

Musculocutaneous Neuropathy

- Injury to musculocutaneous nerve, usually due to trauma / compression
- Musculocutaneous nerve innervates coracobrachialis, biceps, brachialis
- Its terminal portion is pure sensory, the lateral antebrachial cutaneous nerve
  - LAC
- Patient has weakness of elbow flexion, numbness of lateral forearm
- **NCS**
  - Abnormal SNAP to LAC
  - Abnormal CMAP to biceps
- **EMG**
  - Abnormal activity in biceps, brachialis
- **Treatment**
  - Rehab, surgery

Suprascapular Neuropathy

- SSN = C5, C6, upper trunk → suprascapular nerve
- Lies in the suprascapular notch to innervate the supraspinatus, then passes around the **spinoglenoid notch** to innervate the infraspinatus
- Injury is due to trauma, cysts, stretching, upper trunk lesions
  - Often injured in neuralgic amyotrophy (Parsonage-Turner Syndrome)
- Patient has shoulder abduction and / or external rotation weakness

- **NCS**
  - SNAP unavailable
  - Abnormal CMAP to supraspinatus
- **EMG**
  - Abnormal activity in supraspinatus and/or infraspinatus
- **Treatment**
  - Rehab, surgery

Long Thoracic Neuropathy

- C5, C6, C7 → long thoracic nerve
  - "C5,6,7 will get you into heaven on a winged scapula"
- Injury is due to trauma, stretch, compression
- Patient has *medial* winged scapula
  - Lateral winged scapula would indicate trapezius weakness (due to spinal accessory nerve palsy)
- **NCS**
  - SNAP unavailable
  - Abnormal CMAP to serratus anterior
- **EMG**
  - Abnormal activity in serratus anterior
- **Treatment**
  - Rehab (stretch posterior scapular muscles to help facilitate normal protraction)

Brachial Plexus

- The brachial plexus is a web of nerve fibers formed from the C5-T1 nerve roots, that is formed in the neck outside the spine, passes between the anterior and middle scalenes, underneath the clavicle (as cords), and out into the arm as peripheral nerves (terminal branches)
- Roots → Trunks → Divisions → Cords → Branches
- Randy   Travis   Drinks   Cold   Beer
  - C5,C6 → upper trunk → anterior/posterior division → lateral cord → musculocutaneous nerve
  - Divisions are actually not so important...so
    - C5,C6 → upper trunk → lateral cord → musculocutaneous nerve (biceps/brachialis innervation)
- MEMORIZE the upper and lower extremity muscle innervations at the beginning of this lecture, and solving the EMG puzzle of a brachial plexopathy will be a breeze

Brachial Plexus

- Roots: C5, C6, C7, C8, T1
- Trunks: upper trunk, middle trunk, lower trunk
- Divisions: anterior and posterior
- Cords: lateral cord, posterior cord, medial cord
- Branches: musculocutaneous, axillary, radial, median, ulnar (MARMU)

Brachial Plexopathy

- Injury to the brachial plexus occurs usually due to trauma, sports (stretching, compression), radiation, cancer, idiopathic
- The pattern of muscle and cutaneous abnormalities on NCS and EMG will tell you exactly where the lesion is
  - Upper trunk? Lower trunk? Posterior cord? Etc.
- Let's talk about some common brachial plexopathies

Erb Palsy (Upper Trunk Brachial Plexopathy)

- Injured C5, C6 roots/upper trunk
- Typically due to excessive traction forces that stretch the upper trunk out
  - Obstetrical trauma
  - Stinger
- Signs and symptoms
  - Waiter's tip position: arm is adducted, internally rotated, pronated, wrist flexed
  - Weakness of all C5, C6 muscles: deltoid, supraspinatus, infraspinatus, teres minor, biceps, brachialis, brachioradialis, supinator, ECRL, ECRB
  - Sensory loss over lateral arm, dorsolateral forearm
- **EMG/NCS**
  - NCS: abnormal median sensory (C5, C6 fibers), abnormal LAC
  - EMG: abnormal activity and decreased recruitment in the above muscles
- **Treatment**
  - Rehab, splinting as needed, nerve grafting

Klumpke Palsy (Lower Trunk Brachial Plexopathy)

- Injured C8, T1 roots/lower trunk
- Typically due to excessive traction or trauma
  - Fall on adducted arm, being delivered as a baby
- **Signs and symptoms**
  - Claw hand (lumbrical weakness), Wartenberg sign, Froment sign, "OK" sign

- o Weakness of lumbricals, FDS, FDP, FCU, all intrinsic hand muscles
- o Sensory loss of medial arm, medial forearm, and hand
- **EMG/NCS**
  - o NCS: abnormal ulnar SNAP, **normal median SNAP**
  - o EMG: abnormal activity and decreased recruitment in the above muscles
- **Treatment**
  - o Rehab, splinting as needed, nerve grafting

Thoracic Outlet Syndrome (TOS)

- Neurogenic and vascular TOS exist, and both are rare
  - o Neurogenic is most common (compression of nervous structures)
  - o Vascular includes subclavian vessels
- **Vascular TOS:** compression of subclavian/axillary vessels that can lead to upper extremity pulse loss, color changes, cold limb, swollen limb, aching pain
- **Neurogenic TOS:** lower trunk brachial plexopathy (C8,T1 roots)
  - o Lower trunk is compressed by the clavicle and first cervical rib, anterior and middle scalenes, pec minor
  - o Symptoms: pain, sensory disturbance in medial arm, medial forearm, 4th and 5th digits, all worse with overhead activity such as swimming
  - o You can in fact get this kind of symptom pattern from scapular dyskinesis if you end up with a hyperprotracted scapula that squishes the pec minor, clavicle, axillary vessels, and cords of the brachial plexus, leading to neuropathic pain and weakness in whatever cord is affected

Thoracic Outlet Syndrome (TOS)

- **Diagnosis:**
  - o Roos and Adson tests, EMG/NCS
  - o NCS: abnormal ulnar SNAP/CMAP, abnormal median CMAP (median SNAP is normal...why?), MAC
  - o EMG: abnormal spontaneous activity and possibly decreased recruitment of median and ulnar muscles in the hand (lower trunk muscles)
- **Treatment:**
  - o PT (stretching of pec minor and scalenes, strengthening of back muscles), consider surgery for costoclavicular syndrome or tight fibrous band

Parsonage-Turner Syndrome

- *AKA neuralgic amyotrophy, brachial neuritis, idiopathic brachial plexopathy*
- No clear etiology
- Usually unilateral and occurs after a viral illness or surgery

- o Basically some event that triggers the immune system
- Shoulder pain for about 2 weeks, then this gives way to weakness
- **Suprascapular nerve**, long thoracic nerve, AIN are commonly affected
- **EMG/NCS** findings depend on nerve fibers affected
  - o Likely active denervation, decreased recruitment in affected muscles on EMG
  - o Serial EMGs have value for prognosis
- Can resolve on its own; usually within 1-2 years
- **Treatment**
  - o PT

Radiation Plexopathy vs. Pancoast Syndrome

- **Radiation plexopathy:** typically affects C5-C6/upper trunk fibers with a history of radiation (months/years prior). Myokymia on EMG. *No pain.*
  - o Think of this syndrome essentially as painless myokymia
- **Pancoast syndrome:** lung CA that invades upward, thus compressing the C8-T1/lower trunk fibers. Lots of compression and invasion means that this is *painful.* Myokymia is not seen. Invasion can include nearby sympathetic fibers and cause an ipsilateral Horner syndrome.
  - o Think of this syndrome essentially as a painful lower trunk plexopathy

Normal Variations in Upper Extremity Innervations

- **Martin-Gruber Anastomosis**
  - o In some people, median nerve motor fibers cross over in the forearm to join the ulnar nerve
    - ■ Martin-Gruber University → **MGU** → **m**edian-**u**lnar (anastomosis)
  - o This means essentially that the median nerve innervates the ADM and FDI in addition to APB etc.
  - o Ulnar CMAP at the elbow will show a low amplitude when recording over ulnar muscle (e.g. FDI)
  - o Ulnar CMAP will be "repaired"/normal if you stimulate the ulnar nerve at the wrist
  - o So, it looks like there is a conduction block between the elbow and the wrist, but there is not
  - o When you stimulate at the wrist, the median motor fibers have finally joined the ulnar nerve at that point, so you are stimulating all the motor axons that are supplying the ulnar hand muscles
  - o When you stimulate proximally at the elbow, you are not stimulating the median fibers that have yet to contribute to the ulnar innervations, thus you only generate part of the full amplitude

- One thing you can do is record over the ADM/FDI, and stimulate the median nerve at the elbow, to see if you generate a sizeable CMAP
  - If MGA is present, the CMAP amplitude you generate with this will "add up" with the proximal ulnar CMAP to give you your full CMAP from stimulating the ulnar nerve at the wrist

Normal Variations in Upper Extremity Innervations

- **Riche-Cannieu Anastomosis**
  - Median motor fibers in the hand cross over to join the ulnar nerve
  - Essentially now **the ulnar nerve gives motor control to the entire hand**
  - If you record CMAP from APB and stimulate median nerve at the wrist, you will see no CMAP
  - If you record CMAP from APB and stimulate ulnar nerve at the wrist, you will see normal CMAP

EMG is not the confusing beast it wants you to think it is. Break it down into fundamentals and you can understand every concept there is to know about EMGs.

Chapter 17: Lower Extremity Peripheral Nervous System Diseases

List of Upper Extremity Muscle Innervations
- **Muscle Innervations**
- C3, C4; spinal accessory nerve → trapezius, SCM
- C4, C5; dorsal scapular nerve (pre-plexus) → rhomboids
- C5, C6; upper trunk; suprascapular nerve → supraspinatus (then nerve passes through spinoglenoid notch) → infraspinatus
- C5, C6; upper trunk; lateral cord; musculocutaneous nerve → biceps brachii, brachialis
- C5, C6; upper trunk; posterior cord; axillary nerve → deltoid, teres minor
- C5, C6; upper trunk; posterior cord; radial nerve → BR
- C5, C6, C7; long thoracic nerve → serratus anterior
- C5, C6, C7, C8, T1; upper, middle, lower trunk; medial and lateral cord; medial and lateral pectoral nerves → Pec major
- C6, C7; upper and middle trunk; lateral cord; median nerve → PT, FCR
- C6, C7; upper and middle trunk; posterior cord; radial nerve → ECRL
- C6, C7, C8; upper, middle, lower trunk; posterior cord; radial nerve → triceps, anconeus
- C6, C7, C8; upper, middle, lower trunk, posterior cord; thoracodorsal nerve → latissimus dorsi
- C7, C8; middle and lower trunk; posterior cord; radial nerve; PIN → ECU, EIP, ED
- C7, C8; middle and lower trunk; medial and lateral cord; median nerve → FDS
- C7, C8, T1; middle and lower trunk; medial and lateral cord; median nerve; AIN → PQ, FPL
- C7, C8, T1; middle and lower trunk; medial cord; median nerve; AIN → FDP 2,3
- C7, C8, T1; middle and lower trunk; medial cord; ulnar nerve → FDP 4, 5
- C8, T1; lower trunk; medial cord; median nerve → APB, FPB, lumbricals 1,2, opponens pollicis
- C8, T1, lower trunk; medial cord; ulnar nerve → FCU, ADM, FDI, lumbricals 3,4, interossei (3 PADs and 4 DABs)
- **Cutaneous Innervations**
- C5, C6; upper trunk; lateral cord; musculocutaneous nerve; terminates as lateral antebrachial cutaneous nerve (LAC) → skin over lateral forearm
- C8, T1; lower trunk; medial cord; medial antebrachial cutaneous nerve (MAC) → skin over medial forearm

List of Lower Extremity Muscle Innervations
- **Muscle Innervations**
- L2, L3, L4; femoral nerve → quads, iliopsoas
- L2, L3, L4; obturator nerve → adductors; gracilis
- L4, L5; sciatic nerve; deep fibular nerve → tibialis anterior (TA), extensor digitorum longus (EDL)
- L4, L5, S1; sciatic nerve; deep fibular nerve → extensor hallucis longus (EHL), extensor digitorum brevis (EDB)
- L4, L5, S1; sciatic nerve (tibial division) → semimembranosus, semitendinosus, long head of biceps femoris
- L5, S1; sciatic nerve (fibular division) → short head of biceps femoris

- L4, L5, S1; superior gluteal nerve → gluteus medius, gluteus minimus, tensor fascia lata (TFL)
- L5, S1; sciatic nerve; superficial fibular nerve → fibularis longus, fibularis brevis
- L5, S1; sciatic nerve; tibial nerve → tibialis posterior (TP), flexor digitorum longus (FDL)
- L5, S1, S2; inferior gluteal nerve → gluteus maximus
- S1, S2; sciatic nerve; tibial nerve → gastrocnemius, soleus
- S1, S2; sciatic nerve; tibial nerve; medial plantar nerve → flexor hallucis brevis (FHB), abductor hallucis brevis (AHB)
- S1, S2; sciatic nerve; tibial nerve; lateral plantar nerve → abductor digiti quinti pedis (ADQP)
- **Cutaneous Innervations**
- L2, L3; lateral femoral cutaneous nerve → lateral thigh
- L2, L3, L4; femoral nerve; saphenous nerve → medial shin, medial calf
- L4, L5; sciatic nerve; tibial nerve; medial plantar nerve → medial plantar surface of foot
- S1, S2; sciatic nerve; tibial nerve; lateral plantar nerve → lateral plantar surface of foot

Sciatic Neuropathy

- Injury to the sciatic nerve, usually due to trauma, posterior-approach hip replacement, posterior hip dislocation, tight piriformis (piriformis syndrome)
- Injury may preferentially affect tibial or common fibular nerve fibers
    - Usually the common fibular fibers
- Patient typically has weakness in knee flexion, potentially foot drop, along with sensory abnormalities down the back of the thigh and dorsum of foot
    - Essentially weakness in knee flexion +/- ankle and toe mover weakness
- **NCS**
    - Abnormal sural, superficial fibular SNAPs
    - Abnormal EDB, AH CMAP
- **EMG**
    - Decreased recruitment, fibs/sharps in all sciatic nerve muscles; polyphasicity
- **Treatment:** remove offending irritant, stretch piriformis

Common Fibular Neuropathy

- Injury to the common fibular nerve, usually by trauma or stretch (squatting, crossing legs), typically as it wraps around the fibular head
- Patients have foot drop, toe extension weakness, eversion weakness
    - Abnormal sensation to entire dorsum of foot and lateral leg
- Positive Tinel at fibular head
- **NCS**
    - Abnormal superficial fibular and sural SNAPs
    - Normal medial and lateral plantar SNAPs

- o Abnormal EDB and TA CMAP (?conduction block across fibular head)
- **EMG**
  - o Decreased recruitment, fibs/sharps in TA, EHL, EDL, fib longus, fib brevis; polyphasicity
- **Treatment**
  - o Stop offending activity, US-guided decompression, surgical decompression

Superficial and Deep Fibular Neuropathy

- Injury can occur due to tight extensor retinaculum, compression, trauma
- **Superficial Fibular Neuropathy**
  - o Eversion weakness with abnormal sensation over lateral leg and dorsum of foot EXCEPT 1st web space
  - o NCS: abnormal superficial fibular SNAP
  - o EMG: abnormal activity in fib longus and brevis
- **Deep Fibular Neuropathy**
  - o Foot and/or toe drop with abnormal sensation over 1st web space of toes
  - o NCS: normal superficial fibular SNAP
  - o EMG: abnormal activity in TA/EHL/EDL/EDB
- **Treatment**
  - o Remove offending agent, decompress nerve via US or surgery

Tarsal Tunnel Syndrome

- Injury to the tibial nerve as it passes through the tarsal tunnel, usually caused by a tight flexor retinaculum, medial ankle sprain, trauma
- Intrinsic foot weakness, abnormal plantar sensation, +Tinel at medial ankle
- As the tibial nerve passes through the tarsal tunnel, it divides into the medial plantar nerve, lateral plantar nerve, and inferior calcaneal nerve
- Medial plantar nerve
  - o AH, FDB, FHB, 1st lumbrical; medial plantar sensation
- Lateral plantar nerve
  - o ADQP, interossei, all other lumbricals; lateral plantar sensation
- Tarsal tunnel = Tom, Dick, and Very Nervous Harry
  - o Let's draw this out!

Tarsal Tunnel Syndrome

- **NCS**
  - Abnormal medial and lateral plantar SNAPs
  - Abnormal CMAP to AH

- **EMG**
  - Abnormal activity in AH, lumbricals, interossei., ADQP

- **Treatment**
  - Remove compressive irritant (flexor retinaculum surgical release), US-guided decompression

Femoral Neuropathy

- Injury to the femoral nerve (L2, L3, L4), usually due to trauma (catheter stabbing it), accidental during surgery, compression under inguinal ligament, retroperitoneal hematoma, anterior hip dislocation, diabetic lumbosacral plexopathy

- Weakness of knee extensors (knee buckling), abnormal sensation to anterior thigh and medial leg (saphenous nerve)

- **NCS**
  - Abnormal saphenous nerve SNAP and femoral nerve CMAP (rectus femoris)

- **EMG**
  - Abnormal activity in quads

- **Treatment**
  - Remove compression source, surgical release

Saphenous Neuropathy

- Injury to the saphenous nerve, usually due to knee arthroscopy trocar stabbing it on the way in

- Abnormal sensation to medial leg +/- medial knee

- **NCS**
  - Abnormal saphenous SNAP

- **EMG**
  - Normal

- **Treatment**
  - Ensure nothing continues to compress it
  - US-guided decompression
  - Surgical release

Obturator Neuropathy

- Injury to the obturator nerve (L2, L3, L4), usually due to trauma (pelvic fracture)

- Thigh adduction weakness, abnormal sensation to medial thigh

- **NCS**
  - Normal routine SNAPs (sural, superficial fibular)
  - Normal routine CMAPs (EDB, AH)

- **EMG**
  - Abnormal activity in thigh adductors

- **Treatment**
  - Ensure nothing else is entrapping or compressing nerve (bone/scar tissue), rehab, surgical release

Lateral Femoral Cutaneous Neuropathy (LFCN-opathy)

- AKA meralgia paresthetica

- Injury to the LFCN, usually due to tight inguinal ligament, rapid weight loss, diabetes, tight belt, obesity

- Abnormal sensation and burning pain over ovoid patch in anterolateral thigh due to entrapment/irritation of the LFCN

- **NCS**
  - Abnormal SNAP of LFCN

- **EMG**
  - Normal

- **Treatment**
  - Remove compression source
  - Gabapentin, pregabalin, US-guided hydrodissection/block, surgical release

- It is often self-limiting

Lumbosacral Plexopathy

- The lumbosacral plexus involves the L1-S4 nerve roots (ventral rami) that exit the spinal canal and form the web of nerves controlling the lower extremities, known as the lumbosacral plexus

- The **lumbar plexus** involves the L1-L4 nerve roots
  - Anterior division forms the obturator nerve
  - Posterior division forms the femoral nerve and lateral femoral cutaneous nerve (L2, L3)
    - Saphenous SNAP, LFCN SNAP, femoral nerve CMAP

- The **sacral plexus** involves the L4-S4 nerve roots

- o Anterior division forms the tibial nerve
  - ■ Sural SNAP, plantar SNAPs, AH CMAP
- o Posterior division forms the common fibular nerve
  - ■ Superficial fibular SNAP, EDB CMAP
- o Superior and inferior gluteal nerves directly come off the sacral plexus

Lumbosacral Plexopathy

- Injury to the lumbosacral plexus occurs from trauma (pelvic fracture), retroperitoneal bleed, diabetic lumbosacral radiculoplexopathy, neuralgic amyotrophy (AKA Parsonage-Turner Syndrome, just like the brachial plexus), radiation plexopathy, cancer

- Patient has variable weakness and sensory loss depending on which parts of the plexus are affected

- NCS
  - o Variable abnormalities in SNAPs and CMAPs

- EMG
  - o Variable abnormal spontaneous activity and recruitment
  - o Remember, **paraspinals are normal** in all plexopathies!
    - ■ The ventral rami give rise to the plexus, while the dorsal rami innervate the paraspinals

- Treatment
  - o Rehab, address underlying cause, surgery

Diabetic Lumbosacral Radiculoplexopathy

- Injury to the lumbosacral plexus and/or nerve roots due to poor blood sugar control, often in the context of recent weight loss

- **Diabetes often causes a femoral neuropathy** in this manner

- Patient has variable weakness and sensory loss in the lower limbs depending on what parts of the plexus/nerve roots are affected

- NCS
  - o Abnormal lower extremity SNAPs of affected nerves/roots
  - o Abnormal lower extremity CMAPs to affected muscles

- EMG
  - o Abnormal activity in affected lower extremity muscles

- Treatment
  - o Control blood glucose; rehab

Radiculopathy

- Injury to the nerve root(s) exiting the spinal cord via the neuroforamina, usually due to herniated disc (herniated nucleus pulposus), vertebral burst fracture with retropulsion of disc/bony fragments, degenerative spinal stenosis, spondylosis

- Patient has weakness in all muscles served by the affected nerve root (the myotome), even if they have different peripheral nerve innervations
    - *Especially* if they have different peripheral nerve innervations but are from the same nerve root

- Patient also has sensory abnormalities in the affected dermatome
    - Sometimes patients have pure sensory complaints (common), but they can have mixed motor/sensory complaints, or pure motor complaints

- There is no hyperreflexia; there are often depressed reflexes instead
    - If there is hyperreflexia, this is a brain or spinal cord (UMN) lesion, not a radiculopathy

- Imaging (MRI) should show something compressing on the nerve root
    - Herniated disc, osteophytes, stenosis causing narrowing of where the nerve root sits, etc.

Radiculopathy

- **NCS**
    - **Normal SNAPs**
    - Abnormal CMAPs of muscles belonging to affected nerve roots
        - E.g. TA, EDB CMAP will be abnormal in L5 radiculopathy
    - Abnormal H reflex in an S1 radiculopathy

- **EMG**
    - Abnormal activity in all muscles innervated by the injured nerve root
    - Must needle at least 6 muscles in a "root screen"
    - Paraspinals at the affected level will be abnormal
    - Must demonstrate abnormalities in 2 muscles that share the same nerve root, but have different peripheral nerve innervations
        - E.g. C6 radiculopathy showing abnormalities in PT and BR

- **Treatment**
    - Rehab (core and hip girdle strength), medications (gabapentin), ILESI/TFESI, surgery if rapidly progressing weakness or loss of bowel/bladder function or if refractory to the above

Nerve Root Avulsion

- A "tearing off" of the nerve root from its proximal attachment, due to trauma/severe stretch; this has a very poor functional prognosis

- Patient has numbness in affected dermatome, and complete weakness in affected myotome
- MRI can detect nerve root avulsion
- **NCS**
    - Normal SNAPs (because lesion is proximal to DRG, so sensory axons are healthy!)
    - Absent CMAPs
- **EMG**
    - Abnormal spontaneous activity in muscles of the affected myotome; no recruitment whatsoever
    - Abnormal spontaneous activity in affected paraspinals
- **Treatment**
    - Rehab; nerve grafting surgery

Lower extremity EMGs – complete! One final EMG section to go, and you will be…(to be continued…)

Chapter 18: Systemic Nerve and Muscle Disease

Peripheral Polyneuropathy (PN)

- Injury to many different peripheral nerves, usually due to a systemic disease (either inherited or acquired)
- Can be acute onset or gradual onset
  - E.g. Guillain Barre Syndrome vs. length-dependent peripheral neuropathy due to diabetes
- Can be primarily demyelinating or primarily axonal, and can certainly affect both
- Can be primarily sensory or motor, or both (sensorimotor)
- Can be diffuse and symmetric or multifocal and asymmetric
- All of these descriptors are how you should characterize it in your report
- Most PNs are symmetric, and symptomatically and electrodiagnostically *worse distally* than proximally
  - Stocking-glove pattern of symptoms
- The vast majority of PNs will be treated with removal of the offending agent, if possible, and rehab (bracing, PT, OT, etc.)

PN Due to Diabetes Mellitus

- Diabetes causes gradual narrowing of the vasa nervorum (the blood vessels that feed your peripheral nerves), which, over time, causes a length-dependent dying back of the peripheral nerves, starting and the fingertips and toe tips and progressing proximally
- Diabetic PN is the most common form of PN
- Diabetic PN is primarily an axonal process, and is often mixed
- Patient complains of gradual onset numbness and tingling with burning pain in a stocking-glove distribution, finger and toe weakness, often with history of elevated Hgb A1C and poor blood glucose control
- Can see claw toes and hand muscle atrophy on exam, with areflexic achilles reflexes

PN Due to Diabetes Mellitus

- **NCS**
  - Decreased amplitude and prolonged latency of SNAPs
  - Decreased amplitude and prolonged latency of CMAPs
  - Absent F waves
- **EMG**
  - If axonal process, fibs and sharps and decreased recruitment in distal > proximal muscles

- ○ Polyphasicity
- These findings are typically symmetric
- If demyelinating features are present, you may see conduction block and/or increased temporal dispersion on NCS
- Make sure you evaluate at least 3 limbs

PN Due to Other Acquired Causes

- Diabetes is the most common, but many different etiologies exist for acquired PN
- AIDP, CIDP, vitamin B6/B12 deficiency, alcohol toxicity, hypothyroidism, critical illness neuropathy, medication toxicity (e.g. chemotherapy), heavy metals, amyloidosis, CMV, HIV, porphyria, leprosy, uremia
- They will demonstrate similar features as diabetic PN, but there will be key laboratory abnormalities or points in their history that direct the etiology towards something else other than diabetes

Guillain Barre Syndrome (GBS/AIDP)

- AIDP = acute inflammatory demyelinating polyradiculopathy
- Rapidly progressive motor polyneuropathy due to immune system confusing a foreign protein with a protein on your own myelin
- Acute onset ascending paralysis (e.g. over 1-2 days) with ascending areflexia
- All of this is preceded by a recent infection within the past 1-2 weeks
    - ○ GI or upper respiratory infection (campylobacter is very common)
- Paralysis can progress to respiratory compromise
- Diagnose them quickly and give them plasmapheresis/IVIG treatments, and their prognosis is very good

Guillain Barre Syndrome (GBS/AIDP)

- **NCS**
    - ○ The first changes are abnormal (delayed or absent) F waves
    - ○ H reflexes also become abnormal early on
    - ○ F waves and H waves being abnormal early clues you in to the lesion being proximal
        - ■ "Polyradiculopathy"
    - ○ Prolonged latency and reduced amplitude of SNAPs with *sural sparing*
        - ■ Sural nerve is larger, with more myelin than e.g. median and ulnar nerves
    - ○ Prolonged latency, decreased CV, with usually normal amplitude of CMAPs
        - ■ Conduction block, abnormal temporal dispersion

- Distal CMAP amplitude is the key prognostic factor in AIDP
  - If < 20% upper limit of normal, bad prognosis
- **EMG**
  - Decreased recruitment; otherwise normal since no axon loss has taken place
  - However, several weeks after onset, you may see fibs and sharps (active denervation) due to secondary axonal loss, which can occur in AIDP

Chronic Inflammatory Demyelinating Polyradiculopathy

- AKA CIDP; essentially a relapsing-remitting GBS
- Presentation and EDX findings will be similar to AIDP except the symptom progression is much slower in CIDP (months vs. days)
- Patients may recover with plasmapheresis/IVIG/prednisone

Critical Illness Neuropathy (CIN)

- Patients residing in the ICU, typically sepsis/SIRS patients, can develop a great deal of weakness and numbness once they start to recover from their medical illness (e.g. sepsis); commonly this is due to CIN
- This is an axonal sensorimotor polyneuropathy; thus...
- **NCS**
  - Abnormal SNAPs and CMAPs (low amplitude is key feature due to the axon loss)
- **EMG**
  - LDLA, decreased recruitment, fibs and sharps
- **Treatment**
  - Rehab

Inherited Neuropathy

- Genetic diseases (+family history!) that lead to the patient developing a peripheral polyneuropathy
  - This can motor **and** sensory // motor // sensory

Charcot-Marie-Tooth Neuropathy (CMT)

- Has several different subtypes; the most common is CMT1A, a **duplication of the PMP-22 gene**
  - As a young child, gradual distal > proximal weakness with lesser sensory abnormalities
    - Thus, this is a motor and sensory disorder
  - Bilateral foot drop, Champagne bottle legs

- O Deletion of the PMP-22 gene gives you hereditary neuropathy with liability to pressure palsy (HNPP)
- CMT2 gives you an *axonal polyneuropathy*
- **CMT1:** prolonged latency, decreased CV, without conduction block or abnormal temporal dispersion
- **CMT2:** decreased amplitude SNAPs/CMAPs; active denervation/reinnervation on EMG

HIV Neuropathy

- Typically a distal axonal, symmetric sensory > motor polyneuropathy due to HIV/AIDS
- Patient has numbness and tingling with burning in toes and fingers
- **NCS**
  - O Abnormal amplitude of SNAPs/CMAPs
- **EMG**
  - O Abnormal spontaneous activity in distal > proximal muscles
- **Treatment**
  - O HIV medications; rehab

Mononeuritis Multiplex

- Essentially an axonal peripheral nerve injury (e.g. median neuropathy) combined with other single peripheral nerve injuries
  - O For example, left median neuropathy at the wrist, right ulnar neuropathy at the elbow, left radial neuropathy at the elbow, **all in the same patient**
- Can present acutely and asymmetrically with weakness, numbness/tingling
- It is usually due to an underlying vasculitis, which damages axons
  - O Diabetes, Wegener Granulomatosis, polyarteritis nodosa, lupus
- NCS and EMG show abnormalities in the respective peripheral nerves that are damaged, with axonal features generally

Neuromuscular Junction Diseases

- Diseases of the neuromuscular junction, which involve impaired transmission of the action potential across the NMJ synapse due to presynaptic or postsynaptic pathology
  - O Presynaptic = Lambert-Eaton Syndrome (LEMS), Botulism
  - O Postsynaptic = Myasthenia Gravis

Myasthenia Gravis

- Proximal muscle weakness with diplopia that worsens as the day goes on, due to antibodies against postsynaptic acetylcholine (ACh) receptors
- Patients are usually discovered to have a thymoma

- o Thymectomy improves weakness in MG
- Normal ACh quanta are released, but postsynaptic membrane cannot take up ACh
- Labs = +ACh antibodies
- NCS
  - o Normal routine studies
  - o Abnormal repetitive nerve stimulation (RNS)
- EMG
  - o Essentially normal; may see increased jitter and blocking on single-fiber EMG
- Treatment
  - o Thymectomy, pyridostigmine, plasmapheresis/IVIG

Lambert-Eaton Syndrome (LEMS)

- Proximal muscle weakness that is improved with exercise and does not involve diplopia, due to antibodies against presynaptic calcium channels
  - o ACh quanta cannot even be released into the synaptic cleft
- Patients are usually discovered to have small cell CA of the lung
  - o Thus, this is a paraneoplastic syndrome
- NCS
  - o Low amplitude CMAPs
  - o Abnormal RNS
- EMG
  - o Increased jitter and blocking on single-fiber EMG
- Treatment
  - o Rehab; corticosteroids; anticancer therapy, plasmapheresis/IVIG

Botulism

- Dysphagia, diarrhea, diffuse paralysis, respiratory compromise, areflexia due to ingestion of botulinum toxin (home canning, raw meat, raw honey), which cleaves syntaxin/synaptobrevin/SNAP-25, thus inhibiting ACh from being released from synaptic vesicles into the synaptic cleft
- If you can't release ACh onto the muscle membrane, you can't contract the muscle
- Labs: botulinum toxin is detectable in stool or blood
- NCS
  - o Decreased/absent CMAP amplitude
  - o Abnormal RNS
- EMG
  - o Active denervation with decreased recruitment

- ○   Increased jitter and blocking on single-fiber EMG
- **Treatment**
  - ○   Antitoxin; rehab; respiratory support

Repetitive Nerve Stimulation (RNS)

- RNS is a type of NCS performed when the diagnosis is a suspected NMJ disorder
- It involves rapidly stimulating a motor nerve, recording the CMAP over the muscle, and seeing how the CMAP looks when we rapid-fire shock the nerve
- In normal people, the CMAP will look fine
- In NMJ disease, the CMAP amplitude will decrease
  - ○   > 10% decrement in amplitude between 1st and 4th waveforms is positive for NMJ disease
  - ○   In NMJ disease, the safety factor is decreased, making it harder to produce a normal CMAP when ACh quanta are depleted
- RNS can be given at a low rate or a high rate

Low Rate vs. High Rate RNS

- **Low Rate RNS**
  - ○   Muscle is stimulated at 2-3 Hz
  - ○   In NMJ disease, this will cause the aforementioned amplitude decrement
- **High Rate RNS**
  - ○   Muscle is stimulated at 10-50 Hz
  - ○   Calcium builds up in the neuron, which facilitates normal NMJ transmission, and thus, a normal CMAP
  - ○   All NMJ diseases will show a little bit of CMAP repair with this, but LEMS will show a huge increase in CMAP amplitude with this (300%)

Post-Exercise Facilitation and Exhaustion

- **Post-Exercise Facilitation** is essentially the same principle as high rate RNS
  - ○   After low rate RNS is performed and the CMAP has decreased, if the patient performs a maximal contraction in that muscle for 60 seconds, calcium will build up in the neuron and improve NMJ transmission, thus "repairing" the CMAP
- **Post-Exercise Exhaustion** is the idea that the CMAP decreases the more a person exercises overall
  - ○   After a low rate RNS is performed, but the CMAP does not show a decrement, and you still suspect NMJ disease clinically, you can perform another low rate RNS every minute for the next 5 minutes, and one of these tests should show a significant CMAP decrement

- ○ This essentially shows why patients become weaker as the day goes on

Anterior Horn Cell Disease

- Pure motor disease resulting in progressive weakness with normal sensation, due to death of alpha motor neurons (which reside in the anterior horn of the spinal cord)

- Patients typically exhibit LMN signs, but sometimes UMN signs are present as well
  - ○ ALS, PLS, HSP

- **In general**, SNAPs are normal, and latency / CV are also normal, since this is not demyelinating. This NCS picture can be variable.

- Must demonstrate abnormalities in 3 of 4 spinal segments
  - ○ Brainstem, cervical, thoracic, lumbosacral

- SMA, ALS, Poliomyelitis, Post-Polio Syndrome

Spinal Muscular Atrophy (SMA)

- **SMA1: Werdnig-Hoffman Disease**
  - ○ Floppy infant, never sits independently, dies of respiratory failure early

- **SMA2**
  - ○ Weak / floppy 1 year-old, wheelchair as toddler, can sit independently and stand with ADs, dies of respiratory failure

- **SMA3: Kugelberg-Welander Disease**
  - ○ Gradually weakening ~10 year old, can walk independently, normal life expectancy

- Due to mutations in the SMN1 gene

- Labs: elevated CK

- EDX: Normal SNAPs, abnormal CMAPs, LDLA MUAPs with decreased recruitment

- **Treatment:** rehab, **nusinersen, Zolgensma** (onasemnogene abeparvovec-xioi, replaces the mutated SMN1 gene in these patients, creating functional SMN protein)

Amyotrophic Lateral Sclerosis (ALS)

- Degeneration of the anterior horn cells in typically a 60 year-old, leading to progressive pure motor weakness, dysphagia, respiratory compromise without sensory abnormalities

- Poor prognosis with progressive disability and death within a few years

- UMN and LMN signs on exam, including fasciculations

- No bowel or bladder abnormalities

- **NCS**
  - ○ Normal SNAPs; normal CMAPs (due to reinnervation)

- **EMG**
  - LDLA MUAPs, decreased recruitment, fibs and sharps, increased jitter and fiber density
  - Show denervation in 3 of 4 spinal regions (brainstem, cervical, thoracic, lumbosacral)
- **Treatment**
  - Rehab, submaximal exercise, riluzole

Poliomyelitis

- Anterior horn cell degeneration due to poliovirus infection, leading to progressive, pure motor weakness, respiratory compromise without sensory abnormalities
- **NCS**
  - Normal SNAPs
  - Decreased amplitude CMAPs
- **EMG**
  - LDLA MUAPs, fibs and sharps, decreased recruitment
- **Treatment**
  - Supportive

Post-Polio Syndrome

- New-onset progressive weakness in a patient who had fully recovered from polio 15 years ago, with no other etiology to explain the new weakness
- Essentially the anterior horn cells that are remaining after the patient initially recovers from polio just get burnt out from doing all the work and picking up the slack that the dead motor neurons used to carry
  - Imagine 1 motor unit firing at 1 million Hz. It is going to get burnt out and die at some point if it is doing that all your life.
- This is a clinical diagnosis; EMG/NCS is not required
- **NCS**
  - Normal SNAPs
  - Abnormal CMAPs (low amplitude)
- **EMG**
  - **Giant MUAPs**, decreased recruitment, fibs and sharps

Myopathy

- A primary abnormality of muscle fibers (not the peripheral nervous system or NMJ) that leads to variable weakness and abnormalities of muscle contraction
  - Patient is weak with atrophy/hypertrophy and tone/grip issues (hypotonia, myotonia)

- Myopathy can be inflammatory (polymyositis), dystrophic (Duchenne), congenital, metabolic, steroid-induced (steroid myopathy), among other causes

- Muscle biopsy can show Type 1 or Type 2 muscle fiber atrophy
    - Type 2 muscle fiber atrophy occurs in steroid myopathy

- **NCS**
    - Normal SNAPs
    - Abnormal CMAP amplitudes due to atrophied muscles

- **EMG**
    - Small amplitude, short duration, polyphasic MUAPs
    - Early recruitment pattern (i.e. increased recruitment)
    - Sometimes see spontaneous myotonic discharges (divebomber sound)

Dermatomyositis/Polymyositis

- Inflammatory myopathy due to an autoimmune response to virus/cancer

- Proximal hip and shoulder weakness +/- heliotrope rash (dermatomyositis) and Gottron papules (purple patches) over MCPs/PIPs/DIPs

- Type 3 = cancer (e.g. breast/lung) ["Type 3? Not me!"]

- Labs: elevated CK, ESR, LDH; perifascicular atrophy on muscle biopsy

- **NCS**
    - Normal SNAPs and CMAPs

- **EMG**
    - Abnormal (SDSA MUAPs with increased recruitment (early recruitment)

- **Treatment**
    - Corticosteroids, plasmapheresis/IVIG, rehab

Statin Myopathy

- Proximal muscle pain (myalgias) due to statin use, often in setting of CYP450 inhibitors

- **NCS**
    - Normal SNAPs and CMAPs

- **EMG**
    - Normal

- **Treatment**
    - Stop statin, examine medications for those that inhibit CYP450 activity, slowly reintroduce statin, switch to different statin, rehab

Steroid Myopathy

- Proximal muscle weakness due to toxic steroid effect on muscle, usually if patient has been on high doses of steroids for a prolonged period of time at some point in their life
- Causes Type II muscle fiber atrophy
  - EMG generally just analyzes Type I fibers since it takes a maximal contraction to start activating those Type II white fibers
- **NCS**
  - Normal SNAPs and CMAPs
- **EMG**
  - Normal
- **Treatment**
  - Stop steroids if not done already, rehab

Critical Illness Myopathy (CIM)

- Patients residing in the ICU, typically those who have been intubated, given steroids, and been pharmacologically paralyzed, may develop a great deal of weakness and atrophy in both proximal and distal muscles, with **normal sensation**
  - Thus, it is NOT critical illness neuropathy or AIDP
- Labs: elevated CK
- NCS
  - Normal SNAPs
  - Low amplitude CMAPs
- EMG
  - SDSA MUAPS, sometimes fibs and sharps, with normal/early recruitment
- Treatment
  - Rehab (good prognosis, but can take several months to recover)

...unstoppable in all neuro-MSK settings! Which you are now!

Chapter 19: General and Medical Rehabilitation

Gait Cycle

- A person's gait is a rhythmic cycle of **steps and strides** during ambulation

- It is intended to be energetically efficient (i.e. not too taxing)

- There is a normal gait, and there are abnormal gaits that result from various pathologies, typically deconditioning and muscle weakness

- The gait cycle is broken down into the **stance phase** and **swing phase** of the limb
    - **STANCE:** initial contact, loading phase, midstance, terminal stance, preswing
    - **SWING:** initial swing, midswing, terminal swing
    - COG is **5cm anterior to S2 vertebra**, and is at lowest point during loading phase
    - Highest point during midstance

- Typically we spend 60/40 time in stance/swing phase (80/20 single/double limb)

- Running begins once you only have single-limb support

6 Determinants of Gait

- There are 6 things your body does to keep you stable and energetically efficient during your gait; they are:

- Pelvic tilt

- Pelvic rotation

- Pelvic lateral excursion

- Foot mechanisms

- Knee mechanisms

- Knee flexion

Abnormal Gait Patterns

- **Foot Drop ("Steppage Gait")**
    - Cause: dorsiflexion weakness from a variety of causes
    - Foot slaps on the ground during the start of each stance phase
    - Treat with AFO to restore dorsiflexion and smooth rollover gait

- **Trendelenburg Gait ("Gluteus Medius Gait")**
    - Cause: hip abduction weakness, lateral hip pain
    - Weak hip causes contralateral pelvis to drop during stance phase of weak hip (**uncompensated**)
    - Patient throws their torso laterally over the weak hip during stance phase (**compensated**)
    - Treat with hip girdle strengthening, weight loss, pain treatment

- **Genu Recurvatum (knee bending backwards)**
  - Cause: weak or overly active (spastic) knee extensors
  - During or just before stance phase, the knee shoots posteriorly so that it can lock and prevent buckling
  - Can lead to increased knee pain and instability
  - Treat with swedish knee cage (3-point pressure principle of joint correction)

Abnormal Gait Patterns

- **Myopathic Gait**
  - Cause: proximal muscle weakness (E.g. Duchenne Muscular Dystrophy)
  - Hyperlordosis (weak hip extensors), Trendelenburg (weak hip abductors), plantarflexion (tight calf muscles)
  - Treat with bracing (AFO/KAFO/HKAFO) or assisted propulsion (MWC/PWC)

- **Hemiparetic Gait**
  - Cause: stroke, TBI, CP
  - Arm flexion, pronation, wrist flexion, finger flexion, knee hyperextension, excessive plantarflexion
  - Treat with bracing, antispasticity measures (careful not to overtreat and make patient weak)

- **Shuffling Gait (Festinating Gait)**
  - Cause: Parkinson Disease
  - Shuffling feet, very short step lengths, stooped posture, tip-toe pattern
  - Treat with anti-Parkinson medications, deep brain stimulation to subthalamic nucleus (DBS)

Medical Rehab

- "Medical Rehab" consists of rehabilitating patients with significant primary medical disease such as CHF, pulmonary dysfunction, cancer, osteoporosis, burns, or simple aging
- There are some high-yield concepts and facts to know about each of these before you take your boards
- We will cover each of these in this section

Cardiac Rehab

- Before we discuss, let's talk about some cardiac definitions
- Cardiac output: the amount of blood that can pump through the heart in a given "heart sequence"
  - CO = HR x SV
- VO2 max: maximum oxygen consumption a patient can achieve during exercise

- High VO2 max is better!
- VO2 max = CO x AVO2 difference

- MVO2: cardiac oxygen consumption
  - Calculated using the rate-pressure product (RPP)
  - HR x SBP = MVO2

- MET: metabolic equivalent
  - Essentially, how strenuous is an activity relative to baseline metabolic rate
  - E.g. lying flat is 1 MET, and walking on a treadmill is 3 METs

Cardiac Rehab

- Common exercises and their METs
  - Golf is 2 METs
  - Walking at 3 mph is about 3 METs
  - Sex is 5 METs (identical to climbing 2 flights of stairs)
    - No sex for 2 weeks after MI
  - Shoveling snow is 6-7 METs
  - Tennis is 6-8 METs

- We often use the Borg scale to allow patients to report their perceived level of challenge with an activity
  - The Borg scale ranges from 6-20, and we strive for something like 14/15 as a good level of exercise
  - Remember: "Bjorn Borg won Wimbledon on 6/20"
    - High-Yield Note: he did actually win Wimbledon 5 times, but not on 6/20 (it was early July)

Cardiac Rehab

- Patients with cardiac disease, especially heart failure, are often candidates for a cardiac rehab program that serves to increase their function through cardiopulmonary reconditioning
- Cardiac Rehab is delivered in 3 phases
  - Phase 1: inpatient phase (1-14 days)
  - Phase 2: supervised outpatient phase (3-6 months)
    - Patient very closely monitored
  - Phase 3: less supervised outpatient phase
  - Phase 4: unsupervised outpatient, maintenance phase

Cardiac Rehab

- Cardiac rehab benefits patients by reducing deaths from cardiovascular disease, improving exercise ability, tolerance, and fitness, improving blood biomarkers, and improving resting and mid-exercise vital signs

- In general, do not enroll in cardiac rehab if patient has any uncontrolled disease, severe disease, severe pain limitations, or grossly inappropriate vitals
  - See popular board review texts for exhaustive exclusion criteria

- Sometimes we don't know what a patient will be able to tolerate before needing to reduce the METs, so we use graded exercise testing to determine their limits
  - Maximum HR is generally (220 - age), but in cardiac rehab patients we typically use stress testing data to determine this

- Sometimes we use exercise stress tests, pharmacologic stress tests, exercise echocardiogram to determine what their heart can handle
  - In these situations we use treadmills, bicycles, arm-bikes to exercise the patient

Cardiac Rehab

- New York Heart Association Classes of Heart Failure (NYHA 1-4)
- **NYHA 1**
  - Can do anything over 7 METs
  - No real daily limitations or symptoms

- **NYHA 2**
  - Can do anything between 5-7 METs
  - Dyspnea with more than a little activity

- **NYHA 3**
  - Can do anything between 2-5 METs
  - Dyspnea with the smallest activities

- **NYHA 4**
  - Can't really do any activities with comfort
  - **Dyspnea at rest**

Cardiac Rehab

- Patients who have severe heart failure and are candidates for heart transplant typically receive an orthotopic heart transplant, essentially in which the diseased heart is removed and the new heart is placed in its spot

- Once this transplant is completed, the new heart will have a **lower peak HR, higher resting HR**, and **early atherosclerotic disease** (due to being foreign tissue)

Pulmonary Rehab

- Before we begin, let's define some pulmonary terms

- Total lung capacity: total amount of air in the lungs after taking a deep breath (maximal inspiration)
- Vital capacity: the amount of air that can be expelled from the lungs after a deep breath
- Forced vital capacity: same as above, only exhale really hard
- Forced expiratory volume in 1 second (FEV1)
  - The amount of air above that is exhaled in the first second
  - Normally decreases about 30 cc/yr, but in smokers it is much higher
- Minute volume: the amount of air inhaled or exhaled from the lungs in 1 minute
- Residual volume: amount of air in the lungs at the end of a large exhalation
- These are all measured during pulmonary function tests (PFTs)

Pulmonary Rehab

- **We inhale** using the diaphragm chiefly to create negative intrathoracic pressure, which sucks air in
- We also inhale using accessory muscles during exercise or strenuous activity
  - External intercostals, SCMs, levator scapulae, scalenes, pectorals, traps
- **We exhale** using typically nothing but passive air movement, but if coughing or forcefully exhaling, we use abs, internal intercostals

Pulmonary Rehab

- May be beneficial for patients with various forms of lung disease, including restrictive and obstructive diseases
  - Restrictive: lungs do not expand to accept air for gas exchange; decreased lung volumes, difficulty expanding chest wall (obesity, neuromuscular disease, kyphoscoliosis, cervical SCI)
  - Obstructive: increased airway resistance, increased TLC, RV; air trapping
- **Patients benefit from pulmonary rehab chiefly by increasing their AVO2 difference**
  - The peripheral muscles become more conditioned; thus, they take up more oxygen, thus increasing the AVO2 difference
  - Reminder: when doing "cardio", you are really conditioning the peripheral muscles, which improves heart function by allowing the heart to pump less hard and less often

Pulmonary Rehab

- <u>**Medication Options**</u>
- Inhaled steroids to reduce bronchial inflammation
- Inhaled β2 agonists to open the airways (albuterol)

- Inhaled anticholinergics to open the airways (ipratropium)

- Inhaled combination medication (albuterol-ipratropium)

- Mast cell stabilizers (cromolyn sodium)

Pulmonary Rehab

- <u>Therapy and Adjunctive Techniques</u>

- **Postural Drainage**
  - O Patients are placed in various positions of incline or decline to drain obstructive mucus from the various lobes of their lungs

- **Percussion and vibration using hands or machines as part of chest PT**
  - O Can reduce pneumonia incidence and surgical complications

- **CPAP**
  - O Continuous positive airway pressure
  - O Prevents closure of the airway during sleep; **especially useful for OSA patients**

- **Cough assist / coughalator**
  - O Hand-assisted cough (quad cough) can be used by placing hands over patient's abdomen and pushing in when they cough, to help generate expiratory cough force
  - O Coughalator can used to mechanically insufflate and exsufflate the lungs; especially useful for SCI patients

Pulmonary Rehab

- <u>Tracheostomy Tubes ("Trachs")</u>

- Patients with acute respiratory failure, longterm needs for assisted ventilation, and/or obstructive upper airways often benefit from trachs

- The trach is a tube that sits in the trachea and opens the tracheal airway to the air outside the body (basically taking a hollow tube and plunging it through the neck into the trachea)

- **Trachs come in lots of varieties**
  - O **Cuffed:** balloon that inflates, sealing off the upper airway, protecting against aspiration (this means the patient can't talk, since they can't pass air through their vocal cords)
  - O **Uncuffed:** there is no balloon, and so the upper airway **can** pass air
  - O Plastic: cheap, disposable, very common
  - O Metal: durable
  - O Fenestrated: has holes in it that allow air to escape and pass through the vocal cords above

Pulmonary Rehab

- <u>Speaking Valves</u>
- Trachs can have a valve placed over the port on the patient's neck, like a button or cap, that opens to allow air *into the trachea,* and closes to allow exhalation upward, out through the vocal cords and upper airway
- This allows tracheostomy ventilation, yet also proper vocalization
- Only prescribe these if patient can tolerated a deflated cuff, does not have concern for impending decompensation, and is otherwise ready to communicate
- Always start using a speaking valve by ordering a speaking valve trial with a speech therapist
  - Patient and vitals are closely monitored for tolerance through the trial
- When attempting to downsize a trach, always go from cuffed → cuffless before downsizing

Aging

- Causes decreased cardiac output, VO2 max, vital capacity, FEV1, muscle mass, # motor units, peak bone mass starting around age 30, ability to regulate temperature, memory/processing speed, renal GFR, ability to swallow properly,
- Causes **increased fat** (careful with fat-soluble medications)
- With aerobic training, you can increase type IIa fibers, decrease type IIb fibers, and maintain identical number of type I fibers
- With aerobic and strength training, you can increase CO, Hgb, and strength

Cancer Rehab

- This is an expanding field within PM&R, dedicated toward prehabbing and rehabbing patients with a large variety of cancer diagnoses
- The goals are to prevent disability, slow disability, and provide as much comfort and ease of living as possible, all depending on the patient's needs and functional state
- Cancer patients most notably battle **fatigue and pain**
  - Dysphagia is also common

Cancer Rehab

- Common presentations
  - Headache, weakness, seizures → brain tumor (order MRI with contrast)
  - Back pain worse at night → spinal cord tumor (usually thoracic extradural; MRI spine)
  - Extremity pain → primary or metastatic bone disease (NWB, xray, CT, MRI, PET scan)
    - Surgery if at risk for pathological fracture or uncontrolled pain

Cancer Rehab

- Brain Tumors
- Most common primary = astrocytoma (often glioblastoma)
- Most common metastatic = lung, breast, GI
- Children = cerebellar astrocytoma, medulloblastoma
- Patients undergo chemotherapy, radiation, and/or surgery
- Osseous Tumors
- Most common primary = osteosarcoma (usually knee)
- Most common metastatic = lung, breast, prostate, multiple myeloma
- Most are osteolytic
- Prostate CA is osteoblastic

Cancer Rehab

- **Cancer Pain**
    - The WHO developed a cancer pain analgesic ladder for escalating pain needs
    - Step 1: non-opioids, adjuvants
    - Step 2: non-opioids, adjuvants, short-acting opioids
    - Step 3: non-opioids, adjuvants, long-acting/stronger opioids, short-acting opioids
- Non-opioids: acetaminophen, NSAIDs
- Adjuvants: duloxetine, TCAs, gabapentin, pregabalin, etc.
- Short-acting opioids: tramadol, oxycodone, codeine
- Long-acting/stronger opioids: morphine, fentanyl

Pediatric Cancer Rehab

- Leukemia is the most common pediatric cancer
- Brain tumors are the most common **solid** pediatric cancer
    - Pilocytic astrocytoma, medulloblastoma, ependymoma most common
    - Think **posterior fossa tumor** for these
- Rhabdomyosarcoma is the most common peripheral soft tissue cancer
- Osteosarcoma is the most common primary bone cancer
    - Think: the knee

Post-Radiation Syndromes

- **Induced Transient Myelopathy**

- Develops several months after radiation
- Spinal cord sensory neurons are demyelinated
- **Patient recovers** over subsequent several months

- **Delayed Radiation Myelopathy**
  - Develops several months after radiation
  - Sensory and bowel/bladder dysfunction occur
  - **Permanent**

Cancer-Related Lymphedema

- Common after mastectomy as lymphatic drainage system is removed
  - Also occurs after removal of other cancers
- Fluid builds up in the interstitial tissues
- This can cause circulatory problems, cellulitis, poor skin hygiene
- Typically patients develop lymphedema very, very gradually, but it can also occur acutely, quickly, or be related to trauma
- **Grading**
  - **Grade 1: edema reversible with limb elevation**
  - Grade 2: edema of the whole limb, reversible with concentrated effort (stockings, massage, elevation)
  - Grade 3a: edema of the whole quadrant, not reversible, tough tissue, infection common
  - Grade 3b: edema of 2 limbs/quadrants, not reversible, tough tissue, infection common
  - Grade 4: edema more severe in every way than what is in Grade 3b
- Treat with limb elevation, compression, lymphedema massage, PT, OT, diuretics, antibiotics

Burn Rehab

- A burn is a skin injury due to heat, cold, electricity, radiation, chemicals, or friction
  - Usually it is heat-related
- **Heat**
  - Zone of coagulation is dead; zone of stasis is at risk
- **Cold**
  - Direct thermal damage and ischemia
- **Electricity**
  - "Path of least resistance"; nerves, blood vessels are damaged
- **Radiation**

- O   Skin breakdown occurs depending on level of exposure
- Once burned, histamine and prostaglandins cause local vasodilation with edema accumulation
  - O   This is why we give IV fluids to burn patients, to prevent shock

Burn Rehab

- <u>Burn Classification</u>
- **Superficial partial thickness burn**
  - O   Epidermis and part of dermis are damaged
- **Deep partial thickness burn**
  - O   Epidermis and most of dermis are damaged
- **Full thickness burn**
  - O   Epidermis and dermis are totally burned away
- All electrical, inhalational, fracture-related, medically complicated, facial, or perineal burns **must be hospitalized**
  - O   Otherwise hospitalization depends on severity and amount of BSA involved

Burn Rehab

- Use the Rule of 9s to estimate total body surface area (BSA) burned, then give IV fluids and debride burned skin to prevent tissue choking while edema develops
- Topical antibiotics and topical silver are frequently used
- **Rule of 9s** for determining BSA burned
  - O   Head, entire upper extremity = 9% each
  - O   Entire lower extremity = 18% each
  - O   Anterior torso = 18%
  - O   Posterior torso = 18%
  - O   Perineum = 1%

Burn Rehab

- Acute treatment involves fluids and antibiotics as mentioned, but also more directed skin care
- Wound and skin dressings (split or full-thickness skin grafts) are used for deep partial thickness or deeper burns
  - O   Xenographs from different species
  - O   Homographs from cadavers
  - O   Autografts from patient's own donor sites
- Dressings and hydrotherapy are used to debride dead skin
  - O   Very painful and require pretreatment with pain medication

Burn Rehab

- Burns heal by way of inflammation, laying down new collagen, growing new skin, and scar formation with tissue contracture
  - We position the patient optimally to prevent the anticipated contractures
  - Whatever side of a joint a burn is on, the distal part of that joint will want to contract towards the burn
    - E.g. forearm flexor surface burn will lead to wrist flexion contracture
- Optimal position to prevent contractures
  - **Neck extension, shoulder abduction, supination, wrist extension, MCP flexion, PIP/DIP extension, palmar abduction, hip neutral, knee extension, dorsiflexion**
- Remember to watch out for heterotopic ossification (HO)
  - **In burns this is most common at the elbow**
  - **In non-burn patients HO is most common at the hip**

Pediatric Burn Rehab

- Very common cause of accidental death in children, usually by **scalding**
  - **Abuse**
- Rule of 9s applies to children, with adjustments due to their size
  - Head is 18, legs are 14%
  - Every year after 1, subtract 1% from the head, and add 0.5% to each leg
- The same treatment and positioning principles as before apply to children

Bedrest

- Bedrest quickly causes deconditioning in virtually every aspect of the body
- Strength decreases by 1% each day
- Calcium is resorbed from bones no longer performing weight-bearing activity, leading to osteopenia and hypercalcemia
- Immobilization tachycardia occurs
- Decreased lung volumes
- Renal stones
- Constipation
- Skin breakdown

Osteoporosis

- Decreased actual bone mass, leading to weak bones which are prone to fracture
- This is not osteomalacia, which is decreased bone **mineralization**

- ○ With calcium and phosphate, which vitamin D and minerals can improve
- ○ Vitamin D deficiency causes osteomalacia
- **Osteoporosis** is defined as **T-score < under -2.5 on DXA scan**
  - ○ Under 2.5 standard deviations away from average peak bone mass
  - ○ **Normal:** -1 to 1
  - ○ **Osteopenia:** -2.5 to -1
  - ○ **Osteoporosis:** under -2.5
- Risk factors include: white, elderly, female, low BMI, late menses, early menopause, smoking, alcohol, caffeine, lack of weight-bearing activity
  - ○ Female athlete triad is an at-risk population
    - ■ Low BMD, amenorrhea, disordered eating
    - ■ Treat with activity modification, diet, counseling, psychiatry

Osteoporosis

- Treat with bisphosphonates (decrease osteoclast bone-resorption activity; beware jaw osteonecrosis), diet, vitamin D, calcium (typically 1g per day), weight-bearing exercise, calcitonin to decrease acute fracture pain and prevent fractures, estrogen to inhibit osteoclasts, vertebroplasty/kyphoplasty if VB compression fractures occur and are severe enough, bracing

- Screening begins in women at age 65, or younger if risk factors are present

- Fractures in osteoporosis are frequently vertebral body compression fractures and hip fractures

You're a tough, smart doc. And after finishing this chapter, there's nothing General about your Rehab knowledge. Well, actually there probably is now. But you also have very specific knowledge! So that makes you...a very...General, and...Specific...rehab doctor. That's right! You heard it here first!

Chapter 20: Pediatric Rehabilitation

Normal Growth and Development Highlights

- **Manipulate objects** and transfer across midline at 6 months
  - This is when an *upper extremity prosthesis* might be first prescribed (passive mitt)
- **Walk** at one (year old), also the age of rapprochement (exploring close by, then running back to mother)
  - This is when a *lower extremity prosthesis* might be prescribed
- **Primitive reflexes** (moro, fencer, palmar grasp, Babinski) disappear by 8 months
  - Babinski can persist for up to 2 years
- **2 years**, 2-word sentences, 200 words, 2/4 words intelligible (50%)
  - Starts to run
  - Walks upstairs one foot at a time
- **3 years**, 3-word sentences, 3/4 words intelligible (75%)
  - Operates 3-wheel bike (tricycle)
  - Walk upstairs alternating feet
- **4 years**, more complex sentences and word choice, 4/4 words intelligible (100%)

Malformations

- **TORCHS and illicit drugs** cause a variety of fetal malformations
- Toxoplasmosis
- Other (viruses)
- Rubella
- CMV
- Herpes
- Syphilis

Genetic Disorders

- **Down Syndrome**
  - Trisomy 21: upward slanting eyes, simian crease, cardiac disease
- **Turner Syndrome**
  - Missing the second X chromosome, resulting in 45, X karyotype
  - Webbed neck, shield chest, coarctation of the aorta
- **Klinefelter Syndrome**

- Male with extra X chromosome (or female with extra Y), resulting in 47, XXY karyotype
- Tall stature, gynecomastia, small testicles
- All of these can result in some degree of intellectual disability

Congenital Limb Deficiencies

- These occur in utero and result in an incomplete or absent limb, in the transverse or longitudinal direction; historically due to thalidomide or maternal diabetes
- **Left terminal transradial deficiency** is the most common (no limb is present beyond the transradial deficit)
  - **Krukenberg Procedure** is rarely performed
  - Surgically separates the radius and ulna and allows the patient to use them as a pincer to grasp objects (like using chopsticks to pick up food); the advantage is no need for a prosthesis, and patient has sensation in the pincer (which prostheses lack)
- **Fibular hemimelia** is the most common congenital lower limb deficiency
  - **The fibula is absent**, and there is a leg length discrepancy, so some patients have Syme amputation
- **Partial proximal femoral focal deficiency (PFFD)**
  - The femur is short, and patients typically also have fibula deficiency
  - Van Ness Rotation rotates the foot around so that the ankle is effectively the new knee

Pediatric Osseous Defects

- **Club Foot**
  - Severe equinovarus deformity of the foot due to idiopathic cause
  - Cannot walk properly in severe equinovarus deformity
  - Treat with PT, serial bracing, surgery
- **Tibia Vara**
  - Abnormal varus bowing of the proximal tibia
  - Treat with osteotomy of tibia

Pediatric Osseous Defects

- **Developmental Hip Dysplasia / Congenital Hip Dislocation**
  - Malformation of the hip joint (femoroacetabular joint), leading to congenital dislocation of the hip
  - **Galleazzi** test: flex both knees with baby on back; knee is lower on dislocated hip side
  - **Barlow:** with knees in flexion and adduction, apply posterior-directed force to dislocate the hip

- ○ **Ortolani:** relocate the hip and notice the "clunk of relocation" by abducting thighs and applying anterior and medially directed force
  - ○ If any of these tests is positive, patient may have hip dysplasia
  - ○ Ultrasound can assist with diagnosis
  - ○ **Treatment:** Pavlik harness for a few months to avoid hip AVN

Torticollis

- Sometimes babies are born with torticollis due to intrauterine positioning, leading to sternocleidomastoid (SCM) scarring
  - ○ **Torticollis:** excessive sternocleidomastoid (SCM) contraction, resulting in the postural abnormality of head tilting toward that SCM, and chin turning away from that SCM

- **Treatment**
  - ○ PT, ROM of neck and SCM, surgery

Nursemaid Elbow

- Sudden distally directed force on the elbow joint will pull the radial head out of its annular ligament wrapping, causing the radial head to sublux out of the radiocapitellar joint

- This hurts very bad

- **Workup**
  - ○ Xrays will show radial head displacement

- **Treatment**
  - ○ Reduce the subluxation: either hyperpronate the forearm, or flex the elbow while supinating and applying pressure to the radial head

Little Leaguer Elbow

- Similar to VEO syndrome in adults, this is an overuse injury leading to medial condyle traction apophysitis

- **Treatment**
  - ○ Rest, ice, gradual return to activity with correction of throwing mechanics
  - ○ If not treated properly, patient is at risk of impaired bony development of the arm

Osgood-Schlatter Disease

- Overuse injury of the proximal tibias, usually due to excessive jumping or sports activities involving the legs (e.g. basketball) as the patellar tendon pulls on the tibia, leading to tibial tubercle traction apophysitis and fragmentation

- Patients complain of anterior knee pain with activity

- **Workup**

- ○ Xrays are often normal (can sometimes see irregularities of tibial tubercle)
- **Treatment**
  - ○ Rest, ice, gradual return to activity, PT

Transient Synovitis

- Sudden inflammation of the synovium of the hip, leading to sudden-onset hip pain, typically self-limiting
- Commonly a history of URI is present
- **Workup**
  - ○ Xrays normal
  - ○ Labs: elevated ESR
- **Treatment**
  - ○ Rest, ice, NSAIDs, PT
  - ○ Typically self-limiting

Legg-Calve-Perthes Disease

- Not fully explained, but this disease involves hip/groin pain due to the development of AVN of the femoral head
- **Workup**
  - ○ Xrays show femoral head sclerosis
- **Treatment**
  - ○ Rest, hip abduction harness, surgery

Slipped Capital Femoral Epiphysis (SCFE)

- SCFE involves the head of the femur slipping and sliding right off the femoral growth plate, like ice cream sliding off a cone
- Typically occurs in obese adolescent males
- On exam the leg is held in external rotation
- **Workup**
  - ○ Xrays show widened growth plate and femoral head sliding
    - Grade 1 = 0-33% sliding
    - Grade 2 = 34-50% sliding
    - Grade 3 = >50% sliding
- **Treatment**
  - ○ Surgical pinning

Scoliosis

- Abnormal lateral curvature of the spine, usually beginning in adolescence
- This is usually idiopathic, but it can also occur in neuromuscular disease
  - CP, spina bifida, muscular dystrophy
- Dextro vs. levoscoliosis
- Functional scoliosis can also occur, NOT due to skeletal abnormality, but instead for muscular/postural reasons
- When bending forward, the abnormal curve can be viewed from behind patient
- Workup:
  - Xrays: Cobb angle can be measured
- Treatment:
  - Observe a Cobb angle <20°
  - Brace a Cobb angle 20-40° (Milwaukee Brace - 24 hours per day, very restrictive)
  - Surgery for Cobb angle >40° (sooner in neuromuscular disease)

Scheuermann Disease

- This is idiopathic juvenile kyphosis, which can lead to a restrictive lung pattern
- **Workup**
  - Xrays show anterior kyphotic deformity, VB wedging, Schmorl nodes
- **Treatment**
  - PT, TLSO brace, surgery

Group A Strep Rheumatic Fever

- Strep pyogenes (GAS) infection within past few weeks leads to systemic inflammatory reaction
- Jones Criteria for diagnosis include pancarditis, **migratory polyarthritis,** Sydenham Chorea, erythema marginatum, elevated ESR/CRP, evidence of recent GAS infection
- **Treatment**
  - PT, NSAIDs, steroids, all to reduce inflammation and maintain function

Duchenne Muscular Dystrophy (DMD)

- X-linked recessive disease due to gene locus **Xp21 mutation**, leading to practically **no dystrophin** being produced
- This results in a severe progressive myopathy in early childhood in which the normal muscle tissue is replaced by fibrosis, starting with the neck flexors
- Patients walk with a myopathic gait pattern, and lose ambulation ability by age ~10

- O   Gower Sign, calf pseudohypertrophy
- Patients usually use a wheelchair at that time, eventually a power WC
  - O   Scoliosis develops and increases at this time
  - O   Restrictive lung disease develops
  - O   Death (respiratory failure, PNA, cardiomyopathy) as a teenager
- **Labs:** elevated CK; muscle biopsy shows muscle fiber degeneration
- **NCS:** SNAPs normal; CMAP amplitudes low
- **EMG:** myopathic motor units (SDSA, early recruitment, decreased insertional activity)

Duchenne Muscular Dystrophy (DMD)

- **Treatment**
  - O   Submaximal exercise, aerobics, orthoses, steroids, gene therapy eventually
- **Becker Muscular Dystrophy**
  - O   Similar to Duchenne, except the problem is not absent dystrophin, just decreased dystrophin
  - O   Signs and symptoms develop later and are less severe

Myotonia Congenita

- Genetic disorder resulting in myotonia, spasms, and muscle hypertrophy starting at birth, worsened by cold weather
- Patients are unable to smoothly grasp and release (trouble releasing)
- Workup
  - O   NCS: normal
  - O   EMG: myotonic discharges, otherwise normal
- Treatment
  - O   Usually manage without medication

Juvenile Rheumatoid Arthritis (JRA)

- RA in children beginning < 16 years old for at least 6 weeks
- Different subtypes exist: polyarticular, pauciarticular, systemic
- Vast majority are RF-
- **Polyarticular**
  - O   Multiple joints involved; no systemic disease beyond the joints
  - O   Worst prognosis if RF+
- **Pauciarticular**
  - O   <5 joints involved, usually knees or ankles
  - O   HLA-B27+, ANA+

- o Iridocyclitis/uveitis: **ophthalmology referral is mandatory for frequent slit lamp exams**
- **Systemic (Still's Disease)**
  - o Multiorgan system involvement including the joints
  - o Fever, rash, hepatosplenomegaly

Juvenile Rheumatoid Arthritis (JRA)

- Most patients do not develop major disability with treatment
- **Treatment**
  - o PT, strength, ROM
  - o DMARDs (e.g. methotrexate), biologic drugs (e.g. infliximab)
  - o NSAIDs
  - o Corticosteroids

Juvenile Spondyloarthropathies

- Spondylo = spine, so juvenile arthropathies involving the spine
- Ankylosing spondylitis
- Psoriatic arthritis
- Reactive arthritis (Reiter syndrome)
- Enteropathic arthritis (arthritis of IBD)
- SEA syndrome
  - o Sometimes the patient does not demonstrate ANA+ or RF+ on labs, but may develop it later
  - o These children fall into the SEA syndrome
  - o Seronegative enthesopathy and arthropathy

Cerebral Palsy (CP)

- CP is a static, nonprogressive neurologic disease due to a periuterine insult to the brain, resulting in motor, sensory, and/or cognitive deficits
- Major etiologies include intrauterine toxins/teratogens/infections, fetal ICH/anoxic injury, prematurity
- Several types exist: spastic and dyskinetic are most common
  - o Spastic mono/di/tri/tetraplegia depending on # limbs involved
  - o Intellectual disability, sensorineural hearing loss, seizures, bowel/bladder dysfunction
- **Spastic CP** is usually spastic diplegia (essentially a paraplegia)
  - o Typically the child exhibits **spasticity, scissoring, toe-walking, crouch gait**

- **Dyskinetic CP** exhibits movement disorders
    - **Choreoathetosis, ataxia, dystonia**
- **Patient should walk if they sit independently by age 2**

Cerebral Palsy (CP)

- Treatment
    - Involves early intervention program, individualized education program (IEP), education of family, PT, OT, SLP, bracing (typically AFOs or KAFOs), spasticity management, surgery/shunting

Spina Bifida

- Literally, the condition of having a bifid spine
    - Due to failure of the posterior spinal elements to fuse
    - This usually occurs at the L5 or S1 level
- This bifid spine is not a good thing, as spinal cord and/or meninges can herniate through the bony defect and settle just deep to the skin, which leads to deficits of the nervous system
- **Inadequate maternal folate** consumption is a notable risk factor
- Elevated alpha-fetoprotein (AFP) in maternal blood is a screening lab
- Elevated AFP in amniotic fluid is also diagnostic (amniocentesis)
- Fetal ultrasound can also diagnose the neural tube defect
- **Major types of spina bifida** include occulta, myelocele, meningocele, and myelomeningocele ("-cele" means herniation or swelling)

Spina Bifida

- **Spina Bifida Occulta**
    - Posterior spine does not fuse
    - Neither cord nor meninges herniate through the bony defect
    - Hirsute patch on the skin of the back at the level of the defect
    - No major deficits; finding is incidental
- **Myelocele**
    - The cord (myelo) has a swelling just anterior to it
    - Typically lower motor neuron findings of weakness, bowel/bladder dysfunction in lumbosacral elements of spine
- **Meningocele**
    - The meninges herniate posteriorly through the bony defect, forming a large cavity or balloon of spinal fluid with the meninges as the balloon walls
    - Minimal symptoms, as only the meninges protrude through

Spina Bifida

- **Myelomeningocele**
  - Most common form of spina bifida
  - Both cord and meninges protrude through the defect
  - Hydrocephalus (Chiari II) → VP shunt
  - Lumbosacral LMN deficits, bowel/bladder deficits
- **Complications of spina bifida**
  - Tethered cord: cord can "glue" to an area of the spine, resulting in **worsening scoliosis, pain, bowel/bladder dysfunction, weakness** → **MRI spine and surgery necessary to detether cord**
  - Most patients with spina bifida are **allergic to latex** due to frequent health interventions involving latex from a young age
  - Renal disease due to vesicoureteral reflux, UTIs, hydronephrosis, renal calculi, requiring annual renal ultrasound scans for surveillance
- Similar to any SCI patient, prognosis for ambulation varies with the level of motor function remaining

Excellent work! Pediatrics has a lot to memorize, but I know the tips in this chapter will give your memory an edge when it comes to answering test questions and solving clinical pediatric cases.

Chapter 21: Upper and Lower Extremity Prosthetics

Prosthetics

- A prosthesis is a replacement limb or part of a limb, due to amputation, which itself is usually due to trauma or dysvascular disease
    - Upper extremity = trauma
    - Lower extremity = dysvascular disease (PVD, diabetes, factor V Leiden)
- Most commonly these are distal amputations, e.g. transmetatarsal; interphalangeal
- For upper extremity prosthetics, we typically concern ourselves with two main types
    - Body-powered vs. myoelectric
- Lower extremity prosthetics are used for ambulation, and thus do not require the fine control found in body-powered or myoelectric devices

Upper Extremity Prosthetics

- Body-powered prosthesis
    - Consists of a suspension system, socket for the residual limb to fit into, elbow unit, wrist unit, and terminal device
    - It will not necessarily have all of these components, as that depends on the level of amputation of the limb
        - Transhumeral? Transradial? Wrist disarticulation?
    - Let's talk about each of these components in detail

Upper Extremity Body-Powered Prosthetics

- Suspension Systems
    - Necessary so that the prosthesis actually stays on the arm
    - **The Figure 8 harness** is the most common way to do this
        - Loop a strap around the contralateral axilla and wrap it back around to attach it to the prosthesis socket
        - Now the prosthesis is nice and secure, and will not fall off the residual limb
        - The axilla acts nicely as a counterforce for the cable-control action of the terminal device

Upper Extremity Body-Powered Prosthetics

- **Socket**
    - This is the actual hollow tube that the residual limb will fit into
        - It's an encapsulating glove

- All sockets in every prosthesis need to be total contact sockets
  - You will have venous choke points and skin breakdown, warts, etc., if you allow parts of the limb to not remain in contact with the socket wall
    - Exceptions can be made for window cutouts in areas of sensitive skin (bony overgrowth, neuroma, skin breakdown sites)
- Sockets are typically double-walled, consisting of a hard outer socket and a flexible inner socket (which truly encapsulates the limb)
- Sockets **generally** need a separate suspension system as discussed

Upper Extremity Body-Powered Prosthetics

- **Elbow Units**
  - Elbow units are often used if the patient does not have an elbow; i.e. in elbow disarticulations, transhumeral amputees, shoulder disarticulations, and forequarter amputations
  - Elbow units provide flexion and extension action as you might expect

Upper Extremity Body-Powered Prosthetics

- **Wrist Units**
  - The wrist unit connects the terminal device (the prosthetic hand) to the rest of the prosthesis
  - Wrist units in general have 2 types:
    - **Locking wrist:** patient can rotate the wrist around with their normal hand and lock it in place; it will not move from there
    - **Friction wrist:** patient can actually pronate and supinate and perform functional tasks such as doorknob turning; the friction in the wrist can be overcome by heavy objects, however
  - Wrist flexion action can be added, aiding the performance of ADLs such as wiping
  - Bilateral upper extremity amputees may choose electric wrists that aid in rotating the wrists
  - Finally, just distal to the wrist unit is the terminal device (the "hand"), which can be a passive/cosmetic hand, or a functional hand/device/hook/etc.

Upper Extremity Body-Powered Prosthetics

- **Terminal Device**
  - The terminal device is essentially the hand

○ This can be a lot of different things, depending on how functional the patient wants to be (or how functional they actually can be)

○ **Passive fake hand** (for cosmesis)

○ **Hook** (useful for brute force tasks like weight lifting)

○ **Sport-specific prosthesis** (mitt, flipper)

　■ Three jaw chuck pinch (common in body-powered prostheses)

　■ Myoelectric hand (e.g. futuristic cyborg hand, which we'll get to)

○ In general, these all provide no sensation or proprioception, only physical action

Upper Extremity Body-Powered Prosthetics

● **Body-Powered Terminal Devices**

○ These frequently are **three-jaw chuck pincers** that allow the patient to actively grasp objects with force provided by rubber bands

○ **Voluntary-opening** is the most common setup here

　■ The terminal device remains closed at rest, and only by force from the patient will the terminal device actually open and allow the patient to grasp something

○ **Voluntary-closing** is the opposite

　■ This is not as commonly used, because a wide-open prosthesis is a hazard at rest

Upper Extremity Body-Powered Prosthetics

● **How do patients actually control the terminal device?**

○ The suspension system houses cables that run along the length of the prosthesis, all the way to the terminal device

　■ This is often called a **dual cable control system**

○ These cables transmit the proximal forces delivered by the patient all the way through the residual limb and into the prosthesis and terminal device, **thus opening or closing the terminal device at will**

○ The patient does this by performing **biscapular abduction and humeral flexion** to **flex** the elbows into place, followed by biscapular depression and humeral extension to **lock** the elbows into place, followed by this same sequence again to **open or close the terminal device** and ultimately **extend the elbows back down**, resetting the patient back to square one

Upper Extremity Myoelectric Prosthetics

- These are largely the same as body-powered devices, except for the fact that the terminal device is not operated by a cable control system, but instead by muscle contraction of certain remaining muscles in the amputated limb

- Often, **surface electrodes** on the prosthesis inner wall line up exactly with a certain muscle belly

  - When this muscle is contracted, the terminal device will do something

  - E.g. if surface electrode is placed over the wrist flexor group, if patient contracts these muscles, the terminal device will close

  - The opposite can be done for the wrist extensor group in terms of opening the terminal device

Upper Extremity Myoelectric Prosthetics

- Generally these are battery-powered (requiring daily recharging) and **more expensive**

- Remember, they typically have no sensory feedback, which actually is very, very important for performing precise actions

  - This is changing as the years go by and technology progresses

Levels of Upper Extremity Amputation

- Forequarter amputation
- Shoulder disarticulation
- Transhumeral
- Elbow disarticulation
- Transradial
- Wrist disarticulation
- Transcarpal
- Transmetacarpal
- Transphalangeal

Levels of Upper Extremity Amputation

- **Forequarter**

  - Usually necessary due to cancer

  - Difficult situation, as this prosthesis is challenging to operate, and requires special attention towards an acceptable suspension system

  - Patients often opt for a passive prosthesis for cosmetic purposes

- **Shoulder disarticulation**
    - Same as forequarter, although you may see more trauma and infection or compartment syndrome causes here

Levels of Upper Extremity Amputation

- **Transhumeral**
    - Can occur at various lengths (very short, short, standard length)
    - In general, **the longer the residual limb, the better the patient's function**
- **Elbow disarticulation**
    - Surgery is easier and less bloody, and functionally this is a better residual limb than the transhumeral
- **Transradial**
    - The most common congenital limb defect is a left transradial
    - The longer the residual limb, the more pronation/supination remaining

Levels of Upper Extremity Amputation

- **Wrist disarticulation**
    - Full pronation and supination can occur
- **Transcarpal, transmetacarpal, transphalangeal**
    - In general, not as functionally limited as the above levels
    - Often prosthetic fingers will be attached to restore cosmesis

Before Receiving the Prosthesis

- "Prehab" is important!
- Prehab your patients by maintaining strength, ROM of all limbs, wearing a shrinker if necessary, scar mobilization
- Prepare them psychologically for the challenges of losing a limb and using a prosthesis in private and in public
    - Counseling, psychiatry, peer support groups
- Start considering what type of work the patient would like to do with the prosthesis, if any at all
    - Vocational rehab can assist with this

After Receiving the Prosthesis

- Often, inpatient rehab for prosthetic training is indicated and is very useful for a boot camp of getting up to speed with the new prosthesis
    - Learning how to don and doff, operate, perform ADLs, and troubleshoot issues with the prosthesis
- Frequent adjustments to the prosthesis (e.g. socket fit) are required in the initial period, and issues can be identified early on as the patient works daily with the therapists (PT and OT)

Lower Extremity Prosthetics

- Lower extremity amputations are typically due to **dysvascular disease**
    - Diabetes, PAD/PVD, hypercoagulability
    - ABI, dopplers, angiography
- They occur at **various levels** depending on how much limb is viable to be salvaged
- Hemipelvectomy
- Hip disarticulation
- Transfemoral (ideal residual limb shape is **conical**)
- Knee disarticulation
- Transtibial (ideal shape is **cylindrical**; optimal spot to amputate is within proximal 50% of the tibia)
- Ankle (Syme, Boyd, Pirogoff)
- Foot (Chopart, Lisfranc, Transmetatarsal, Transphalangeal)

Amputation Planning

- Prehab the patient, maintaining strength and ROM of all limbs
- During surgery, the surgeon will perform either a myoplasty or a myodesis so that the transected muscles don't simply hang in place
- **Myoplasty**
    - Muscles are sutured to each other
    - Easier surgery
- **Myodesis**
    - Muscles are sutured into the bone
    - More stable surgical result
    - Not suitable in severely dysvascular patients, as this will not heal properly

After Receiving the Prosthesis

- As with upper extremity prosthetics, the patient will require prehab and rehab with their prosthesis

- They will need to wear a shrinker for essentially 24 hours per day for a prolonged period of time until postoperative edema has resolved (this can take months, but is well under a year), and then they can have their definitive prosthesis fabricated

- Scar mobility/massage, proper moisturization, sweat management, are all important

- They will need to learn how to don and doff it, troubleshoot issues, and perform ADLs with it

- This is best done in an inpatient rehab setting

- Now let's talk about exactly *what* the lower extremity prosthetics entail

Lower Extremity Prosthesis Components

- Very similar to upper extremity prosthesis components

- Suspension system

- Socket (total contact fit)

- Knee unit (for transfemoral and above)

- Pylon (also known as shank)

- Foot

- Cosmetic cover

- Which components the patient is prescribed depends on their **K level**, which is determined by the physician after taking a thorough history and performing a physical exam

K Levels

- These were introduced by Medicare in an effort to curb inappropriate prescriptions

- They describe how functional of an ambulator a patient is projected to be

- **K0** = nonambulatory - "zero prosthesis"

- **K1** = limited household ambulator, fixed cadence

- **K2** = unlimited household; limited community ambulator; fixed cadence

- **K3** = unlimited community ambulator, variable cadence

- **K4** = high impact activities; sports, variable cadence

Energy Cost of Ambulation

- With the K Levels in mind, always think about the cost of ambulation for the patient

- For amputees, their energy cost of ambulation is a certain % above normal patients'

- **Traumatic Amputees**
  - Unilateral TT - bilateral TT - unilateral TF - bilateral TF
  - 20%   40%   60%   200%

- **Dysvascular Amputees**
  - Essentially just double the above values and you are in the right ballpark

Lower Extremity Prosthesis Components

- **Suspension System**
  - **Transfemoral**
    - Suction system with a one-way expulsion valve that expels air from the socket, creating a good suction seal and total contact within the socket
    - Locking pin
    - Suspension belt that wraps around contralateral side
  - **Transtibial**
    - Suction suspension
    - Locking pin
    - Supracondylar cuff: this is essentially a thigh cuff wrapped around the thigh above the level of the femoral condyles, providing suspension by clinging to the thigh

Lower Extremity Prosthesis Components

- **Socket**
  - **Transfemoral**
    - **Ischial containment socket** is preferred. This is a narrow ML socket. Double-walled construction with flexible inner socket and outer shell. It maintains a little thigh adduction and flexion to place the abductors and extensors in a mechanically advantageous stretched position. Weight is borne by the ischia, the natural "sit bones".
    - **Quadrilateral socket** is an older socket that is narrow AP, wide ML.
  - **Transtibial**

■ Double-walled construction with flexible inner socket and outer shell to provide total contact fit which is vital to maintaining a healthy limb and good suspension

■ These sockets are often referred to as "patellar tendon-bearing sockets" - PTB - which we will discuss on the next slide

Lower Extremity Prosthesis Components

● Pressure within the transtibial socket must be distributed over pressure-tolerant areas, with relief areas for pressure-intolerant areas

● **Pressure-tolerant areas**

○ Patellar tendon (hence the name), medial tibial flare, medial tibial shaft, anterior tibial muscles, fibular shaft, popliteal fossa

● **Pressure-intolerant areas**

○ All other areas are pressure-intolerant

Lower Extremity Prosthesis Components

● **Knee Units** (for transfemoral or above)

○ In general these attempt to mimic a human knee by allowing it to bend when not in the middle of weight-bearing, and not allowing it to bend while weight-bearing is taking place, so that it does not buckle

○ These are typically single-axis or polycentric

■ **Single axis:** the knee bends freely along one axis of flexion/extension. Simple, reliable, cheap, durable knee. Patient must supply muscular power to maintain extension, but this is assisted by using a manual lock or constant friction system to disallow free bending/collapse

■ **Polycentric:** more closely mimic the human knee; multiple axes of rotation are present; more complicated, heavier, more expensive; often use hydraulics (air or fluid) to accomplish natural bending and weight-bearing of the knee

Lower Extremity Prosthesis Components

● **Specific Knee Units**

○ Manual Locking

○ Constant Friction

○ Stance Control

○ Polycentric

○ Fluid-controlled: air (pneumatic), oil (hydraulic)

○   Microprocessor

Lower Extremity Prosthesis Components

● **Pylon**

     ○   This is also known as the shank

     ○   It is basically the "tibia"

     ○   Not much variation here; it does its job of bearing weight

Lower Extremity Prosthesis Components

● **Foot**

     ○   SACH (solid ankle, cushioned heel)

         ■   Useful in Syme amputation for flat surfaces

         ■   Simulates natural rollover motion of the foot on the ground

     ○   Single Axis Foot

         ■   Flat surfaces; 1 axis of rotation (plantar-dorsi)

     ○   SAFE (stationary ankle, flexible endoskeleton)

         ■   Useful for uneven surfaces

     ○   Multiaxis Foot

         ■   Allows motion in plantar-dorsi and inversion-eversion planes for uneven surfaces

     ○   Energy-storing Foot

         ■   Pylon and foot are one unit formed in a C shape to allow compression and energy storage, like a spring

     ○   Specialty Foot

         ■   Sports or work-specific feet are available, such as a flipper prosthesis for swimming

Complications of Lower Extremity Amputations

● **Phantom sensation**

     ○   The feeling that the amputated part of the limb is still there, generating sensory signals; not usually painful or bothersome

● **Phantom pain**

     ○   Neuropathic pain in the limb distal to the amputation site, i.e. in the "ghost" limb; this is painful and is usually treated with gabapentin, pregabalin, TCAs, SNRIs

○ Not usually a chronic issue; usually does not persist beyond 6-12 months

- **Nociceptive pain**

  ○ Can be due to a large number of causes: skin conditions, bone spurs, HO, infection/cellulitis, fresh incision, poor skin mobility, neuroma

Complications of Lower Extremity Amputations

- **Bone spurs**

  ○ May develop due to poor surgical technique; can be a source of nociceptive residual limb pain

- **Heterotopic ossification**

  ○ May occur, typically in a traumatic amputation

  ○ Dx: xrays, US, alk phos, ESR/CRP/CK, bone scan

  ○ Treatment: bisphosphonate, indomethacin, surgical removal once HO matures

Complications of Lower Extremity Amputations

- **Skin problems**

  ○ Poor socket fit can lead to areas of **venous choking**, which causes verrucous hyperplasia (warts)

    ■ This happens if part of the socket is too tight around the limb, and the rest of the distal limb hangs in place without being in contact with the socket wall, essentially choking the distal limb's venous return

    ■ Treatment is typically adjusting the number of sock ply worn by the patient, or fabricating a new socket

  ○ Folliculitis, boils, abscesses, tinea corporis may result from poor hygiene and excessive moisture/sweating

    ■ Treat with oral antibiotics, antifungals, I&D, antiperspirants as needed

Troubleshooting Gait Abnormalities

- **Transfemoral**

  ○ Abducted, circumducted gait, or vaulting on the prosthetic side

    ■ Causes: prosthesis is too long; inappropriate sizing of socket walls, providing discomfort; abduction contracture; patient does not trust the knee to bend properly and stabilize them; poor suspension; knee unit not flexing properly

Troubleshooting Gait Abnormalities

- **Transtibial**
  - **Excessive varus moment**
    - Causes: foot is set too far medially; socket is too abducted
  - **Excessive valgus moment**
    - Causes: foot is set too far laterally; socket is too adducted
  - **Excessive knee flexion**
    - Causes: not enough friction built into the knee unit; too much dorsiflexion in the foot; weak quads; socket placed too far anteriorly; foot placed too far posteriorly; knee flexion contracture
  - **Excessive knee extension**
    - Causes: too much friction built into knee unit; too much plantarflexion in the foot, weak quads (recurvatum), socket placed too far posteriorly; foot placed too far anteriorly

Pediatric Prosthetics

- Often these are due to congenital limb deficiencies, the most common of which is a **terminal left transradial** deficiency
  - Note, it is a deficiency, not an amputation; thus, the child does not have phantom sensation/pain, and does not "suffer" the loss of a limb
  - Parents must accept the prosthesis in this case, as must the child
- Children are prescribed a prosthesis as soon as they would be using that limb in normal development (i.e. 6 months for upper extremity prosthesis, and around 12 months [sometimes earlier] for lower extremity prostheses)
  - The prosthesis is replaced every year until age 5, then every 18 months until age 12, then every 2 years until age 21

Pediatric Prosthetics

- Children rapidly grow, so sometimes an onion socket design is used, in which layers can be removed from the socket as the child grows
- Bony overgrowth can occur in acquired amputations, and this is different from heterotopic ossification
  - Distal bone grows too fast and becomes very sharp and pointy
  - Surgery may be required

Think of this chapter as a prosthesis for your…prosthetics…knowledge. You know, that doesn't sound as cool as I thought it would. You understand prosthetics now. You get the idea.

Chapter 22: Orthotics

Orthotics

- An **orthosis** is a brace used largely to promote proper positioning of a limb, stabilize a joint, relieve pain, stretch spastic muscles, or promote function

- In order to achieve stable manipulation of a joint, **the 3-point pressure principle** must be followed

- Most orthotics are plastic, rubber, metal, or some combination

  ○ Thermoplastics can provide a more custom fit

- We will cover orthoses in a (mostly) head-to-toe format

Cervical Spinal Orthosis

- This is used to stabilize the cervical spine in cases of spinal fracture or SCI

- **Halo vest**

  ○ Used in unstable C-spine fractures (e.g. type 2 dens fracture), this is the most restrictive cervical orthosis; it is essentially a ring halo around the patient's head, that is bolted down to the skull via 4 long pins; the halo is connected to the vest that the patient wears securely

  ○ Often patients graduate from this to a rigid cervical collar

- **Minerva Jacket**

  ○ This is a CTO that can be used in place of the Halo vest for unstable cervical fractures; useful since it is not invasive like the Halo vest is

  ○ Disadvantageous because it is a large, cumbersome, unappealing, stiff jacket

Cervical Spinal Orthosis

- **Sterno-Occipital Mandibular Immobilizer (SOMI)**

  ○ Uses bars that connect to one another from the sternum, occiput, and mandible to limit cervical ROM

  ○ Can be used for stable cervical fractures

- **Rigid cervical collar / Philadelphia collar**

  ○ Provides control of the neck in all panes, but not as well as the Halo vest

  ○ Wraps around the jaw and back of the head, extending down onto the chest to prevent motion in all planes

- **Soft Cervical Collar**

  ○ Soft foam collar that does not restrict motion; simply provides a kinesthetic reminder for patients to maintain neck in proper posture

      O   Patients can become dependent on them, so use sparingly

Thoracolumbosacral Orthosis (TLSO)

- The TLSO stabilizes the TLS spine in cases of spinal fracture, SCI, or postoperative after spine surgery

- **Jewett Brace / CASH Brace**

  - O   Jewett and CASH braces prevent hyperflexion of the TL spine in cases of vertebral body compression fractures

  - O   CASH brace is less cumbersome

- **Taylor Brace / Knight-Taylor Brace**

  - O   Used similarly to Jewett and CASH braces, these have straps that wrap over the shoulders (like overalls), with the brace covering the abdomen and low back, promoting an upright spine posture

- All of these TLSOs help to "brace the core" which is similar to weight lifters using an abdominal lifting belt; i.e. the TLSO increases intraabdominal pressure which allows forces to be transmitted into the abdomen, and NOT through the spinal column

Scoliosis Bracing

- **Milwaukee Brace**

  - O   This is essentially a CTLSO that consists of a neck ring supported by bars from the thoracolumbosacral region, which allows for forces to be generated to correct a scoliotic spine and maintain it in correct position

  - O   Must be worn at all times except for bathing, until skeletal maturity is reached

  - O   Indicated if bracing is indicated for scoliosis (i.e. scoliotic curve is 20-40 degrees)

Soft Lumbosacral Bracing

- **Lumbar Corset**

  - O   Soft, flexible brace that doesn't really do much; indicated for myofascial low back pain/strain

  - O   Use with caution, as it can promote atrophy and dependence

Upper Extremity Orthoses

- Upper extremity orthoses are very common in patients with TBI, stroke, and SCI, who often also have spasticity in their upper extremities

- Proper positioning of a limb is vital to prevent contractures in patients with spastic muscles

- This is achieved with braces that not only provide stretch of spastic muscles, but place pressure over tendons of spastic muscles, manipulating spastic reflexes, and have inherent properties of their materials that manipulate spasticity of the muscles it is in contact with

- Let's talk about various upper extremity orthoses that are used

Specific Upper Extremity Orthoses

- **Resting hand splint**
  - Useful in spasticity or burn patients with the goal of preventing contractures
  - Hand is maintained in the intrinsic plus position (slight wrist extension, MCP flexion 70-90 degrees, thumb in palmar abduction, PIPs and DIPs in extension)

- **Tenodesis orthosis**
  - Used often in SCIs involving an NLI of C6 (patient has some wrist extensor power, but nothing in C7 roots or below – i.e. no hand/finger control)
  - This brace extends the wrist, thus approximating the fingers with the thumb, allowing a more functional grasp to be achieved by the patient

Specific Upper Extremity Orthoses

- **Universal cuff**
  - This is a hand splint that allows a soft hollow tube to rest in the patient's palm, allowing them to pick up objects and manipulate them (e.g. fork/spoon)

- **Opponens orthosis**
  - Immobilizes the thumb to allow healing (often ligamentous injuries)
  - This can be a long opponens orthosis which extends further up the wrist to prevent radial or ulnar deviation of the wrist (useful in arthritis conditions that cause wrist deviations)

Specific Upper Extremity Orthoses

- **Swan neck and Boutonniere ring splints**
  - Correct the deformities of the above conditions by counteracting the positions of the diseased joints

- **Finger orthoses**
  - Maintain PIPs and/or DIPs in extension, promoting ligament and fracture healing

- **Shoulder-elbow-wrist-hand orthosis**
  - This is akin to the lower extremity HKAFO
  - Support of the hand, wrist, elbow, and shoulder joint via a complete housing apparatus allows the patient to feed themselves as long as they have grade 2/5 elbow flexor and shoulder girdle musculature

Ankle-Foot Orthosis (AFO)

- An AFO is a calf and foot brace that generally prevents plantarflexion and assists in a normal rollover gait and foot clearance
- Useful in spasticity (stroke, TBI, SCI, CP) involving excessive plantarflexion tone and dorsiflexion weakness
- It is also useful in flaccid ankle weakness
- Usually the foot plate extends just beyond the metatarsal heads, but if the toes are in spastic flexion, then the foot plate may extend all the way to include the toes
- AFOs are usually plastic (can be off-the-shelf or custom-molded AFO)
- Metal AFOs consist of metal bars that provide limb control
  - Used in cases of fluctuating limb volume, skin sensitivity, or skin breakdown
- Plastic AFOs come in 3 primary types
  - Rigid, semirigid, and posterior leaf spring (PLS)

AFO Pins and Springs

- Pins and springs can be added to the anterior or posterior channels of the AFO in order to prevent (pins) or assist (springs) plantarflexion or dorsiflexion
- Pins in the **anterior** channel of the AFO will prevent dorsiflexion
- Springs in the **anterior** channel will assist plantarflexion
- Pins in the **posterior** channel will prevent plantarflexion
- Springs in the **posterior** channel will assist dorsiflexion

Plastic AFOs

- **Rigid AFO**
  - Also called solid AFOs; these prevent any motion at the ankle or foot. We use these in cases of severe spasticity to prevent any ankle or foot motion

- **Semirigid AFO**
  - A little bit of ankle motion is allowed in order to facilitate a normal gait pattern, but, as the ankle muscles are weak, structural support is still needed

- ○ Useful if there is not severe spasticity requiring the control of a rigid brace
- **Posterior leaf spring (PLS)**
  - ○ Allows the most ankle plantar/dorsi ROM and mediolateral ROM
  - ○ Useful in flaccid foot drop with no spasticity
  - ○ The posterior channel spring serves as dorsiflexion assistance

Knee-Ankle-Foot Orthosis (KAFO)

- A KAFO extends the AFO design all the way up to include the knee
  - ○ Useful if patient has impaired muscular control of the knee (e.g. paraplegia, CP)
  - ○ The KAFO has straps that wrap it around the thigh for anchoring, a hinge joint mechanism to bend with the patient's knee, and bars connecting the knee area to the AFO
- Often the hinge joint is actually offset posteriorly to the patient's knee; **this causes the line of gravity to fall anterior to the knee**, tending to lock it in extension
  - ○ This is useful in patients with quadriceps weakness whose knees would otherwise buckle
- **Bail locks**
  - ○ Automatically lock the KAFO in extension when the knee is extended, allowing the patient to get up and walk without having to "do anything"
  - ○ To unlock the knee, the patient pulls up on a lever near the knee; the drawback is that this bail lock can accidentally be pulled (bail locks are contraindicated for bilateral use)
- **Drop locks**
  - ○ "Drop down" to lock the knee on their own via gravity; the drawback is that sometimes it requires participation from the patient

Hip-Knee-Ankle-Foot Orthosis (HKAFO)

- Useful for entire lower extremity weakness, including the hip girdle
- Extends the KAFO all the way up to include the hip
- HKAFOs come in different flavors, one of which is the reciprocal gait orthosis
- The RGO is an HKAFO that houses cables that join the two lower extremities' forces together; i.e. when one leg advances, the other extends backwards, to simulate a normal gait pattern
  - ○ Thus, the RGO requires intact hip flexion power

Knee Braces

- Knee orthosis provides stabilizing forces to the knee joint alone; i.e. this is not a KAFO (there is no ankle piece)

- Soft knee braces can be bought over the counter and generally provide kinesthetic reminders (e.g. for proper patellar tracking in PFPS or knee OA) and perceived sense of a more stable knee

- Harder braces are often used following bony or ligamentous injury

- **Lennox-Hill Derotation Orthosis** is used following an ACL tear to prevent further stress to the ligament

- **Swedish Knee Cage** is used to prevent genu recurvatum using the 3-point pressure principle

- **Patellar Tendon-Bearing Orthosis** uses uprights from the ankle area to transmit forces into the patellar tendon so it can share the load of weight-bearing; this reduces forces in the foot and ankle (useful in foot and ankle fractures)

Shoes

- Shoes are made up of the toe cap, vamp, 2 hind quarters, sole, and heel

- Variations can be made in the materials and dimensions of these structures to allow a custom fit

- The sole has an insole and an outsole

- The "ball" of the foot is the widest part of the sole

- The heel absorbs impact from walking/running

    o Heel wedges can be used to treat knee OA pain

- Soles and heels can be excavated to provide pressure relief

- Pads can be added for comfort

Shoes

- **Custom insoles** can provide custom pain relief and support

    o Plantar fasciitis, bone spurs

- **Rocker bar**

    o An arch placed posterior to the metatarsal heads that permits a nice, smooth, rollover gait, places the pressure on the MT shafts to relieve the MT heads

    o Metatarsal bar is similar but shorter

- **Heel or sole wedges/flares** can promote/prevent inversion or eversion

Orthotics! The physiatrist's secret toolbox. The keys to the toolbox are now yours.

Chapter 23: PM&R Pharmacology

PM&R Pharmacology

- PM&R utilizes a wide variety of medications to help functionally enable patients

- A strong understanding of these medications and their uses is a powerful asset to every PM&R physician, resident, and medical student

Nociceptive Pain Medications

- **Opioids**
  - Naturally derived or synthetic chemicals that reduce pain by binding to mu, kappa, and delta receptors located in the CNS
    - Natural opioids are **morphine and codeine**
    - Synthetic opioids are all the rest
      - Oxycodone, hydrocodone, hydromorphone, buprenorphine, fentanyl, tramadol, methadone
  - Binding to mu, kappa, delta lowers presynaptic Ca^{2+} influx and increases postsynaptic K^+ transport, which together reduce synaptic action potential transmission of central pain fibers
  - The different receptors do different things
    - Mu_1 = pain reduction
    - Mu_2 = respiratory depression, nausea/vomiting
    - Kappa = respiratory depression
    - Delta = pain reduction

Nociceptive Pain Medications

- **Opioids**
  - **Indications**
    - Acute trauma, postsurgical pain
    - Severe, uncontrolled pain
      - Grey area
  - **Contraindications**
    - Patients with addiction/abuse history or risk
    - Uncomplicated arthritis
    - "Back pain"
    - Chronic pain - not effective; produces dependence
  - **Notable Side Effects**
    - Respiratory depression and death, hypogonadism/low testosterone
    - Do NOT combine with benzodiazepines, as this may cause respiratory depression and death
      - Have the patient pick one

Nociceptive Pain Medications

- **Specific Opioid Medications**
    - ○ **Morphine**: short or long-acting pain control
        - ■ Acute pain: 5-10 mg PO Q4H PRN
        - ■ Chronic/long-acting pain control: extended-release morphine: 15-60 mg PO Q12H
    - ○ **Oxycodone**: short-acting pain control (sometimes long-acting)
        - ■ Acute pain: 2.5/5/10 mg PO Q4-6H PRN
    - ○ **Fentanyl:** long-acting pain control
        - ■ Acute pain: 25-200 mcg TRANSDERMAL Q72H
    - ○ **Hydromorphone:** short-acting pain control
        - ■ Acute pain: 2 mg PO Q4-6H PRN
    - ○ **Codeine:** short-acting pain control
        - ■ Useful for aborting intractable tension headaches, especially in neurologic disease (stroke)
        - ■ Acute pain: 15-30 mg PO Q4H PRN

Nociceptive Pain Medications

- **Specific Opioid Medications**
    - ○ **Methadone:** chronic pain agent
        - ■ Useful for treating chronic pain or weaning off chronic opioid addiction
        - ■ Methadone is also an NMDA antagonist, the effect of which helps to treat pain
            - ● Ketamine is also an NMDA antagonist
        - ■ Chronic pain: 2.5-20 mg PO Q8-12-24hrs
    - ○ **Buprenorphine:** opioid-detoxification agent
        - ■ Useful for helping opioid-dependent patients wean off opioids
        - ■ Has mixed agonist-antagonist activity
        - ■ Often combined with naloxone for opioid detoxification/weaning
        - ■ Chronic pain/detoxification: 8-16 mg SL DAILY
            - ● Dose varies depending on induction vs. maintenance doses, and the individual
    - ○ **Naloxone:** opioid antagonist
        - ■ Useful for opioid weaning/detoxification, and for reversing respiratory depression
        - ■ Opioid reversal: 0.2-2.0 mg IV (divided in boluses)

Nociceptive Pain Medications

- **Specific Opioid Medications**

- ○ **Tramadol**
  - Sort of a "step down" from opioids
  - Mu agonist and serotonin-norepinephrine reuptake inhibitor
  - Milder pain medication than most opioids
  - Can cause sedation
  - 25-100 mg PO Q4-6H PRN

Nociceptive Pain Medications

- ● **Basic analgesic and antipyretic**
  - ○ **Acetaminophen**
    - Acetaminophen works by inhibiting prostaglandin production (COX enzyme) in the CNS, thus inhibiting pain and fevers centrally
    - There are no GI side effects when compared to NSAIDs
    - Useful for mild pain
    - 500-1000 mg ONCE-QID (total max daily dose of 3 or 4 g, depending on setting)
      - Dose is limited by potential hepatotoxicity

Nociceptive Pain Medications

- ● **Nonsteroidal Anti-Inflammatory Drugs (NSAIDs)**
  - ○ NSAIDs work by inhibiting COX-1 and/or COX-2 enzyme
    - COX enzymes convert arachidonic acid to inflammatory mediators like **prostaglandins**
    - Thus, if you inhibit COX, you inhibit prostaglandin production
      - Thus, reduced inflammation → reduced inflammatory pain
    - COX-1 produces prostaglandins that protect the stomach lining
      - Thus, NSAIDs reduce these protective prostaglandins and cause gastric ulcers
      - To circumvent this, meloxicam and celecoxib have been developed to act more selectively on COX-2, thus protecting the stomach (theoretically)
    - NSAIDs are effective for acute, inflammatory pain
      - Tendonitis, bursitis, arthritis, tenosynovitis, tension headaches, myofascial pain
      - Not advisable to use them chronically, due to risk of gastric ulcers and renal disease
      - Contraindicated if history/presence of gastric ulcer or AKI/CKD
    - Sometimes we ask patients to hold NSAIDs prior to interventional procedures so that proper healing and pro-inflammatory response can take place postprocedurally

Nociceptive Pain Medications

- **Specific NSAIDs**
  - **Ibuprofen**
    - 200-800 mg PO Q4-6H PRN
  - **Naproxen**
    - 220-500 mg PO Q12H PRN
  - **Indomethacin**
    - Useful for heterotopic ossification (HO) treatment
    - 25-50 mg PO BID-TID
  - **Diclofenac**
    - Useful as a topical gel/cream for superficial MSK pain (greater trochanter, hand/wrist, shoulder)
    - 1% gel 2-4 g TOPICALLY QID PRN
  - **Celecoxib**
    - COX-2-selective NSAID that is theoretically gastroprotective relative to the other NSAIDs
    - 100-200 mg PO BID
  - **Meloxicam**
    - COX-2-selective NSAID that is theoretically gastroprotective relative to the other NSAIDs
    - 7.5-30 mg PO DAILY

Topical Pain Medications

- **Topical fentanyl**
  - Patch form discussed in opioids section

- **Topical diclofenac**
  - Discussed in NSAIDs section

- **Topical lidocaine**
  - **Lidocaine gel**
    - Comes in various % concentrations, usually 2%
    - Useful for bowel and bladder care in SCI patients
    - Thin spread TOPICALLY BID-TID PRN
  - **Lidocaine patch**
    - Comes in various % concentrations, usually 4-5%
    - Useful for MSK pain, especially neck, back, and shoulder pain; can be cut and divided
    - 1 patch TOPICALLY DAILY

- Don't forget ice and heat!

Neuropathic Pain Medications

- Neuropathic pain medications work by various mechanisms and are useful for pain related to neurologic dysfunction
    - Stroke, TBI, SCI, CRPS, phantom pain, neuralgia

Neuropathic Pain Medications

- **Specific Neuropathic Pain Medications**
    - **Amitriptyline**
        - TCA that inhibits reuptake of serotonin and norepinephrine in the CNS
        - It has antidepressant and anti-neuropathic pain properties
        - It can prolong the QT interval
        - It is anticholinergic as well, so it can cause dry mouth, urinary retention, constipation
        - It can contribute to serotonin syndrome
        - 25-200 mg PO QHS (QHS as it can cause somnolence)
    - **Gabapentin**
        - Blocks L-type Ca^{2+} channels in the CNS (originally developed as an antiseizure medication)
            - This inhibits synaptic transmission
        - Can cause somnolence, mood stabilization (useful for TBI/mood disorder)
        - 100-1200 mg PO DAILY-TID (900 mg PO QID also possible) (3600 mg maximum daily dose)
    - **Pregabalin**
        - Same mechanism as gabapentin
        - FDA-approved for diabetic neuropathic pain, postherpetic neuralgia, fibromyalgia
        - 50-200 mg PO BID-TID

Neuropathic Pain Medications

- **Specific Neuropathic Pain Medications**
    - **Duloxetine**
        - Serotonin-norepinephrine reuptake inhibitor (SNRI)
        - Has both antidepressant and antineuropathic pain properties
        - FDA-approved for diabetic peripheral neuropathic pain and fibromyalgia
            - Along with pregabalin
        - Useful in mood disorder patients (e.g. depression) with neuropathic pain
        - 30-60 mg PO DAILY

- ○ Venlafaxine
    - SNRI
    - Similar indications and effects as duloxetine
    - 25 mg PO TID (IMMEDIATE RELEASE) / 37.5-75-150 mg PO DAILY (EXTENDED RELEASE)

Neuropathic Pain Medications

- **Specific Neuropathic Pain Medications**
    - ○ **Carbamazepine**
        - Inhibits Na⁺ channels on neurons, thus preventing signal transmission along nerves
        - Useful for trigeminal neuralgia in particular
        - Also useful as a mood stabilizer (TBI patients)
        - 100-200 mg PO BID-QID
    - ○ **Injectable anesthetic**
        - With or without steroid is useful for peripheral nerve-related neuropathic pain
        - The anesthetic works by inhibiting pain fiber sodium channels
        - The steroid works by inhibiting PLA2, thus inhibiting production of arachidonic acid, and by direct neuronal membrane inhibition, thus inhibiting pain fiber signal transmission
    - ○ **Capsaicin**
        - Hot pepper chemical that depletes substance P (substance P helps transmit pain signals)
        - Topical capsaicin is useful for intractable neuropathic pain over a small area (e.g. hand)
            - CRPS, SCI
        - Apply smallest amount necessary to cover the affected area 1-4 times DAILY

Anti-Inflammatory Medications

- Anti-inflammatory medications generally include NSAIDs and corticosteroids
- **NSAIDs** as discussed in pain medication section
- **Corticosteroids**
    - ○ Inhibit PLA2 enzyme; thus, arachidonic acid is not produced
        - Thus, inflammatory mediators (prostaglandins) are not produced from arachidonic acid
        - Thus, inflammation and inflammatory pain are reduced
    - ○ Useful in reducing **inflammatory pain**
        - HNP causing radiculopathy / radiculitis

- Bursitis, tendonitis, acute osteoarthritis or rheumatoid arthritis
  - ○ Can be taken orally or injected
    - Phonophoresis, iontophoresis can be used for transdermal steroids, but this is not common
  - ○ **Prednisone**
    - 5-60 mg PO DAILY
  - ○ **Triamcinolone, methylprednisolone, dexamethasone**
    - Dexamethasone is nonparticulate (used in spinal injections)

Antispasticity Medications

- Antispasticity medications work by inhibiting mechanisms that cause spasticity to take place
  - ○ Spasticity: velocity-dependent increase in resistance to passive stretch of a muscle
  - ○ Graded on Modified Ashworth Scale (MAS) as grades 1-4 (review spasticity section for details)
- Generally they work centrally to inhibit the spinal cord motor reflex arc
  - ○ Except dantrolene which works peripherally on the sarcoplasmic reticulum of muscle fibers
- This means that generally they cause sedation, and generally they also lower the seizure threshold
- Specifically we will discuss baclofen, diazepam, tizanidine, dantrolene, and botulinum toxins

Antispasticity Medications

- **Specific Antispasticity Medications (all listed are FDA-approved)**
  - ○ **Baclofen** = centrally acting $GABA_B$ agonist
    - $GABA_A$ = binding here increases presynaptic Cl^- influx into the neuron
    - $GABA_{B1}$ = binding here inhibits presynaptic Ca^{2+} influx into the neuron
    - $GABA_{B2}$ = binding here increases postsynaptic K^+ conductance out of the neuron
      - All of these actions inhibit synaptic transmission and the firing of neurons
      - If you can't fire neurons, you can't fire muscles to make them contract
      - **"CLACK"**
        - ○ Chloride, Calcium, Potassium
        - ○ Cl^-, Ca^{2+}, K^+
    - Side effects: sedation, respiratory depression, lower seizure threshold
    - Withdrawal risk: patient becomes "itchy, bitchy, and twitchy"

- Clearance: renally cleared, so use lower doses in patients with CKD or select another agent
- Dose: usually start 5 mg PO QHS, titrating up to 20-30 mg TID
- See SCI and Interventional PM&R sections for intrathecal baclofen pump discussion

Antispasticity Medications

- **Specific Antispasticity Medications (all listed are FDA-approved)**
  - **Diazepam** = centrally acting GABA$_A$ agonist (Cl$^-$ channel activator)
    - **CLACK!**
    - Side effects: sedation, respiratory depression
    - Withdrawal risk: seizures
    - Clearance: hepatically cleared, so use caution with liver disease
    - Dose: 2-10 mg PO TID

Antispasticity Medications

- **Specific Antispasticity Medications (all listed are FDA-approved)**
  - **Tizanidine** = centrally acting α_2 agonist (as is clonidine) which inhibits the spinal reflex arc
    - Side effects: sedation, respiratory depression, lower seizure threshold
    - Withdrawal: HTN, tachycardia, anxiety, worsened spasticity
    - Clearance: hepatically cleared, so **check LFTs prior to dosing,** and monitor 1x per week for several weeks to ensure stability before spreading LFTs out over time
    - Dose: usually start 2 mg PO QHS, then increase up to 12 mg TID (36 mg/day)
  - **Dantrolene** = peripherally acting, binds to the ryanodine receptor on the sarcoplasmic reticulum in muscle cells, which then inhibits the influx of Ca^{2+} from the sarcoplasmic reticulum into the cell
    - No Ca^{2+} means the muscle can't contract
    - Side effects: sedation, weakness
    - Withdrawal: worsened spasticity
    - Clearance: hepatically cleared, so **check LFTs prior to dosing,** and monitor 1x per week for several weeks to ensure stability before spreading LFTs out over time
    - Dosing: start 25 mg PO BID, titrating up to 400 mg/day (BID or TID dosing)

Antispasticity Medications

- **Specific Antispasticity Medications**
  - **Botulinum toxin injections**

- Botulinum neurotoxins inhibit the presynaptic syntaxin, synaptobrevin, and SNAP-25 proteins which are full of neurotransmitters about to be released into the synapse
- By cleaving these proteins, the toxin prevents neurotransmitter (ACh) from being released
  - This process is called **chemodenervation**
- Thus, neurons can't fire, muscles can't contract, and you are paralyzed
- By focally injecting this into select muscles, we can locally paralyze individual muscles, such as those that are too spastic
- Black box warning of distant toxin spread, which may cause dysphagia, respiratory depression, so use with caution with existing motor neuron disease such as ALS
- "3 days, 3 weeks, 3 months" (onset, peak, duration of action)
- Botulinum toxin is especially useful if you want to avoid systemic medications with systemic side effects
- Dose: many brands exist, and the dosage per muscle depends on the brand, size of the muscle, degree of spasticity in each muscle, and risk factors for dysphagia and side effects

Bowel Medications

- These are used to help regulate the GI tract and stool output with the goal of producing regular, daily, soft bowel movements (BMs)
- They are most frequently used in the SCI population, but are very common among all inpatient rehab patients, and are also used in the outpatient setting

Bowel Medications

- **Specific Bowel Medications**
  - **Docusate**
    - Stool softener that helps to "grease the groove" so that bowel movements slide easily and the patient does not have to strain, which can lead to hemorrhoids and increased abdominal and intracranial pressure (via the Valsalva maneuver)
    - It allows water and fat into the stool to make it softer
    - 100 mg PO DAILY-BID-TID
  - **Senna**
    - Senna is a **s**timulant that irritates the bowel wall to promote peristalsis
    - (187 mg tabs) 2 tabs PO DAILY (give ~8 hours before intended BM)
  - **Polyethylene glycol (PEG)**
    - Osmotic laxative that pulls fluid into the bowel lumen, promoting urgency of BM
    - It is considered a mild laxative
    - 17 g PO DAILY

Bowel Medications

- **Specific Bowel Medications**
  - Lactulose
    - Intended as a treatment for hepatic encephalopathy, as it traps NH_3 in the bowel, thus allowing it to be excreted instead of accumulating in the body
    - Lactulose, however, is also a powerful osmotic laxative
    - Lactulose is usually reserved in cases of constipation resulting in no BM for typically 2+ days
    - Always a good idea to rule out bowel obstruction with a KUB (abdominal xray) before ordering lactulose
    - 20-80 g PO ONCE (give ~2-4 hours before intended BM)
  - Bisacodyl
    - Rectal wall irritant that is used to stimulate rectal propulsion and evacuation of stool bolus
    - Using a gloved finger and lidocaine jelly, suppository is inserted deep into the rectum with rectal wall stimulation in a 360° sweep to dilate the rectal wall and encourage it to evacuate
    - 10 mg PR DAILY/PRN

Bladder Medications

- These are commonly used in the SCI population to treat UMN bladder (spastic bladder; the goal is to calm the bladder down)

- UMN bladder is small and spastic, and the detrusor muscle squeezes spastically with even the smallest (100 cc) amount of urine filling the bladder

- This leads to incontinence and increased UTIs

- As noted in the SCI section, the bladder empties via cholinergic parasympathetic pathway (pelvic nerve), and it stores urine via noradrenergic sympathetic pathway (hypogastric nerve)

- Thus, our bladder medications are aimed at either stimulating or inhibiting these pathways to achieve our desired result

Bladder Medications

- **Specific Bladder Medications**
  - Oxybutynin
    - Strong anticholinergic that inhibits cholinergic activity upon muscarinic ACh receptors in the bladder wall, thus blocking the ability of the detrusor muscle to squeeze the bladder spastically
    - Useful in SCI with UMN injury and spastic bladder
    - Anticholinergic side effects of **dry mouth, constipation, sedation**

- 5 mg PO TID (immediate release) / 10 mg PO DAILY (extended release)
  - Tolterodine
    - Same mechanism as oxybutynin
    - Tends to be gentler than oxybutynin in both bladder effect and side effects
      - "Little old lady" version of oxybutynin
    - 2 mg PO BID (short-acting) / 4 mg PO DAILY (long-acting)

Bladder Medications

- **Specific Bladder Medications**
  - **Mirabegron**
    - β^3 agonist that acts selectively on the bladder wall β receptors, theoretically focusing action there and reducing untoward side effects
    - It acts NOT via the parasympathetic cholinergic pathway (as the previous drugs did), but instead on the sympathetic noradrenergic pathway
    - By stimulating β^3 receptors, mirabegron promotes storage in the bladder
    - 25 mg PO DAILY
  - **Bethanechol**
    - Pro-cholinergic medication that is intended to increase bladder detrusor activity and, thus, promote bladder emptying by stimulating muscarinic ACh receptors in the bladder wall
    - Useful in LMN (cauda equina) bladder injuries (failure to empty)
      - These patients typically demonstrate overflow incontinence
    - Cholinergic side effects (runny nose, hypersalivation, diarrhea)
    - 10-25 mg PO TID-QID

Bladder Medications

- **Specific Bladder Medications**
  - **Tamsulosin**
    - α_1 blocker that acts in the urinary bladder neck to inhibit the sympathetic (noradrenergic) action upon the bladder neck, which normally results in squeezing of the bladder neck and, thus, promotion of urine storage (or, prevention of bladder emptying)
    - Thus, tamsulosin opens up the bladder neck to facilitate adequate emptying of the bladder
    - Many SCI patients have detrusor-sphincter-dyssynergia (DSD) in which the detrusor contractions and the bladder neck contractions/relaxations are not timed properly, and the detrusor ends up squeezing while the bladder neck is tight, thus causing vesicoureteral reflux into the ureters

- Tamsulosin opens up the bladder neck so that when the detrusor squeezes, urine goes OUT instead up UP into the kidneys
  - 0.4-0.8 mg PO DAILY (can cause hypotension, so often given at bedtime)

Anticoagulation

- Blood thinners that are used on most inpatient rehab patients to prevent DVT/PE

- The general rule of thumb is to keep patients on anticoagulation (AC) until they are consistently ambulating >150 feet at a time

- Incomplete SCI patients are usually on AC until IPR discharge

- Complete, uncomplicated SCI patients: 8 weeks

- Complete, complicated SCI patients: 12 weeks
  - Age > 60, cancer diagnosis, long bone fracture, history of DVT

- If unable to use AC due to risk of bleeding, plan for IVC filter

Anticoagulation

- **Specific Anticoagulation Medications**
  - **Heparin**
    - Rapid-acting agent that activates antithrombin 3, which then inhibits Factor Xa
    - Rapid onset, rapid reversal with protamine sulfate (if needed)
    - Risk of heparin-induced thrombocytopenia (HIT), so monitor platelets
    - 5,000 units SQ Q8-12H (prophylaxis) / drip form (treatment of DVT/PE)
  - **Enoxaparin**
    - This is a low molecular weight heparin
    - Also reversed with protamine sulfate
    - 30-40 units SQ DAILY (prophylaxis) / 1 mg/kg body mass SQ BID (treatment)

Stroke/TBI Medications

- Stroke and TBI patients often draw from the same medication array

- Most of these medications are cognitively acting to improve arousal (via increased dopamine) or stabilize an uninhibited mood

- In general for neurostimulation, much of the research is still being developed

Stroke/TBI Medications

- **Specific Stroke/TBI Medications**

- ○ **Amantadine**
    - ■ Neurostimulation agent used to improve arousal
    - ■ Can lower the seizure threshold
    - ■ Originally developed as an anti-influenza drug, but it was found to also potentiate dopamine (DA) release in the brain, thus theoretically increasing arousal
    - ■ Useful in patients whose low arousal levels are inhibiting their therapy participation
    - ■ Also useful in patients who exhibit behavioral problems ("agitation") due to poor energy levels
    - ■ 100 mg PO DAILY-BID (last dose should be at noon, or you will keep them up at night!)
- ○ **Modafinil**
    - ■ Exact mechanism unknown; thought to be related to dopamine reuptake inhibition
    - ■ Could conceivably lower the seizure threshold
    - ■ 100-200 mg PO QAM

Stroke/TBI Medications

- ● **Specific Stroke/TBI Medications**
    - ○ **Methylphenidate**
        - ■ Norepinephrine-dopamine reuptake inhibitor
        - ■ Useful for ADHD, narcolepsy, and neurostimulation in stroke/TBI
        - ■ Does not lower the seizure threshold (i.e. does not increase seizure risk)
        - ■ 10 mg PO BIDAC (dose can vary) / 20 mg PO DAILY (long-acting form)
    - ○ **Donepezil**
        - ■ Cholinesterase inhibitor; thus, promotes ACh accumulation in the brain (cholinergic)
        - ■ May be useful as a neurostimulant especially in anoxic brain injury
        - ■ 5-10 mg PO DAILY
    - ○ **Fluoxetine**
        - ■ SSRI, useful in treating depression associated with stroke and also **enhancing motor recovery from stroke**
        - ■ 20 mg PO DAILY

Stroke/TBI Medications

- ● **Specific Stroke/TBI Medications**
    - ○ **Levetiracetam**
        - ■ Anticonvulsant (antiseizure) medication that is generally well tolerated

- Useful for seizure disorder and early posttraumatic seizure prophylaxis in TBI patients
- Exact mechanism unknown
- Can cause sedation and mood stabilization
- 500 mg PO BID x7 days (seizure prophylaxis)

○ **Phenytoin**

- Anticonvulsant as above; exact mechanism unknown - potentially Na^+ channel blockade
- Literature supports use of phenytoin for early PTS prevention, but we tend to use levetiracetam as above due to favorable side effect profile
- Can cause sedation and mood stabilization
- 150 mg PO/IV Q8H (this varies by patient weight)

Stroke/TBI Medications

● **Specific Stroke/TBI Medications**

○ **Valproate**

- Voltage-gated Na^+ channel blockade; mechanism not fully understood
- Useful as antiseizure medication and mood stabilizer in "agitation"
- Can cause excessive sedation; can check with blood level
- 10-15 mg/kg/day (max 60 mg/kg/day)

○ **Carbamazepine**

- Inhibits Na^+ channels on neurons, thus preventing signal transmission along nerves
- Useful for trigeminal neuralgia in particular
- **Also useful as a mood stabilizer (TBI patients)**
- 100-200 mg PO BID-QID

Psychiatric Medications

● In PM&R, the profound disabilities of our patients often lead to significant psychiatric disease, including depression and adjustment disorder

● Many different medications, therapy, and counseling are useful for these patients

● SSRIs, SNRIs, TCAs (as discussed)

● Sleep and appetite-stimulating medications can help (next section)

Sleep Medications

● **Specific Sleep Medications**

○ **Trazodone**

- Serotonin reuptake inhibitor that is used as a combination antidepressant-sleep aid

- Risk of serotonin syndrome., especially if used in combination with other serotonergic drugs
- 25-150 mg QHS PRN

- **Mirtazapine**
  - Increases central serotonergic and noradrenergic activity
  - Useful to increase appetite, improve mood, and serve as a sleep aid
  - 15-30 mg PO QHS

Neuromuscular Disease Medications

- Neuromuscular disease medications in general do not cure the disease, but they do improve lifestyle and function to a degree
- In particular we will discuss pyridostigmine, riluzole, and nusinersen

Neuromuscular Disease Medications

- **Specific Neuromuscular Disease Medications**
  - **Pyridostigmine**
    - Anticholinesterase drug; thus, ACh activity is potentiated
    - Useful for **myasthenia gravis** patients in which anti-ACh-R antibodies block the postsynaptic ACh channels from binding ACh
    - With pyridostigmine, all the extra ACh in the synapse can overwhelm these antibodies and allow the patient to actually fire their neuromuscular synapses as intended
    - 600 mg PO DAILY GIVEN IN DIVIDED DOSES / 180-540 mg PO DAILY-BID (long-acting)
  - **Riluzole**
    - Blocks glutamate action in the CNS (has other blockade effects as well)
    - Useful for **prolonging survival by a few months in ALS patients**
    - Dosing per neurologist

Neuromuscular Disease Medications

- **Specific Neuromuscular Disease Medications**
  - **Nusinersen**
    - Alters the splicing activity of SMN2 gene so that it produces more SMN protein
      - SMA patients are deficient in SMN protein due to mutations in their SMN1 gene
      - Without SMN protein (survival motor neuron protein), motor neurons die
    - FDA-approved for treating **spinal muscular atrophy (SMA)**
    - Shown to improve motor function and ambulation

■ Administered intrathecally

Injectable Medications

● Like the title implies, these are any medications that you will push through a needle during interventional procedures

● IV medications will not be discussed here, and are not very common in PM&R in general

● Injectable medications in this section include local anesthetics, steroids, regenerative "medications" such as platelet-rich plasma (PRP) and prolotherapy, and botulinum toxins

● Accuracy is markedly increased with ultrasound guidance (can also combine with EMG guidance for neurotoxins)

Injectable Medications

● **Specific Injectable Medications**
  ○ **Local anesthetics (lidocaine, bupivacaine, ropivacaine)**
    ■ Local anesthetics are Na$^+$ channel inhibitors, thus inhibiting action potential transmission
    ■ Rapid onset (they do burn upon injection, however)
    ■ Very useful for subcutaneous and "pathfinder" numbing action as your needle finds its way to its target (consider for more difficult injections or those with risky targets)
    ■ Useful for diagnostic injections (e.g. facet joint injections, medial branch blocks, etc.)
    ■ Anesthetics suspended in fluid come in a variety of concentrations
    ■ Each has a different duration of action
      ● Lidocaine 1-3 hours
      ● Ropivacaine 4-6 hours
      ● Bupivacaine 4-8 hours
    ■ Monitor for allergies or toxicity; consider pre-treatment with diphenhydramine and prednisone
    ■ Note: local anesthetics are toxic to tenocytes (ropivacaine less so)
    ■ Depending on the target to be injected, sometimes it is most prudent to not use any anesthetic

Injectable Medications

● **Specific Injectable Medications**
  ○ **Corticosteroids**
    ■ As discussed previously, perform direct inhibition of pain fiber neuronal membranes, and inhibit PLA2 enzyme to decrease arachidonic acid and

inflammatory mediator production, thereby reducing inflammatory pain mediators

- Useful for more long-lasting pain relief (aim for 2-3 months of relief)
    - Joints, tendonitis, bursitis, radiculopathy/radiculitis, neuralgia/neuritis
- Corticosteroids are essentially toxic and do nothing to actually repair tissue; their job in injections is to reduce pain long enough for physical therapy to get the patient "over the hurdle" of strength and pain so that they can now become more functional instead of trying to "rehab through the pain"
- Side effects: hyperglycemia, osteoporosis, metabolic syndrome, thin skin, hypopigmentation of skin
- Methylprednisolone, triamcinolone, dexamethasone

Injectable Medications

- **Specific Injectable Medications**
    - **Platelet-Rich Plasma (PRP)**
        - PRP is generated when a patient's blood is drawn, spun in the centrifuge machine, and the platelet-rich layer is drawn up into a syringe
        - This is an out-of-pocket expense in America ($500-1000 per blood draw)
        - Data are gradually being generated demonstrating its utility in regenerating cartilage and repairing partially torn or diseased tendons and ligaments
        - Sometimes used in combination with other regenerative techniques such as percutaneous needle tenotomy or tendon scraping procedures for tendonosis
    - **Prolotherapy**
        - Dextrose is diluted down to a 25% dextrose solution (diluted using sterile water/normal saline/local anesthetic) and injected into damaged tissue (joint, tendon, ligament, over cartilage or labrum)
        - This is an out-of-pocket expense in America (approximately $125 per injection – varies widely)
        - Cheaper than PRP
        - Also used in combination with other regenerative procedures, as above

Forget calling the pharmacy with questions. We'll just call you! But uh, do call the pharmacy with questions.

Chapter 24: Interventional PM&R

Interventional PM&R

- Consists of the various procedures that PM&R physicians and subspecialists are trained to do

- Procedures are hard! That's ok.

- Repetition, repetition, repetition

- Everybody is terrible at procedures for a while before getting good

- We will discuss **common** palpation-guided, ultrasound-guided, EMG-guided, and fluoroscopic procedures in detail

- This is not meant to be a comprehensive procedural guide; there are excellent guides available for more depth. Refer to a procedure atlas for your procedural skills development and reference.

Interventional PM&R

- **Palpation-guided ("blind") approach**
  - Anatomical surface landmarks are used to achieve accuracy and hit your target

- **Ultrasound-guided approach**
  - The target, "innocent bystander structures", and needle are visualized during the procedure to achieve accuracy

- **EMG-guided approach**
  - Used in botulinum toxin injections, this is very useful to identify active motor units in a spastic muscle, and to ensure the muscle you want to inject truly is spastic (as evidenced by the abundance of firing motor units when in the muscle)
  - Needle is a modified EMG needle that is hollow, allowing for passage of medication through the needle

- **Fluoroscopic approach (xray guidance)**
  - Xray beam is used to target various joints, generally for axial injections

Interventional PM&R

- **Clean technique**
  - The needle tip only touches sterilized surfaces before piercing alcohol-swabbed skin
  - Nonsterile gloves are used
  - All injected medications are always sterile in the vial
  - This is not full sterile technique
  - For most injections this is sufficient to reliably prevent infection
  - For ultrasound, sterile gel and sterile probe cover are still used

- **Sterile technique**
  - All equipment is dropped onto a sterile field, typically a tray stand with a sterile cover placed over it
  - The patient's skin over the injection site is cleaned with sterile cleaning solution
    - Typically chlorhexidine x3, applied in concentric expanding circles
  - A sterile field (sterile towels) is placed over the skin, leaving only the injection site exposed
  - Sterile gloves are used throughout the procedure
  - Sterile gowns are typically not worn
  - For ultrasound, sterile gel and sterile probe cover are used

Palpation-Guided Injections

- **Trigger Point Injection**
  - Trigger points are hyperirritable bands of tight muscle and fascia tissue that produce local numbness and tingling along with local + radiating pain and tightness
    - When palpating there may be a local twitch response of the muscle
    - **Trigger point:** physician can feel it, and it radiates pain outward
    - **Tender point:** physician can't feel it, and it does not radiate pain outward
  - Physical therapy and postural re-education are the mainstays of treatment
  - Sometimes trigger point injections are useful to "get them over the hump"
  - Typically trigger points are located in the **upper back and neck musculature**
  - **Procedure**
    - Palpation-guided, clean technique
    - 25+ gauge 1-1.5 inch needle
    - Dry needle or small volume (2-3 cc total) of local anesthetic +/- corticosteroid
    - Identify trigger point and mark it with skin indentation, then wipe skin with alcohol swab
    - Make multiple needle passes through each trigger point, fanning the needle out to different spots at that location

Palpation-Guided Injections

- **Shoulder (glenohumeral joint) Injection**
  - Indicated for known GHJ arthritis, failing PT and analgesics
  - Palpate the **coracoid process** medial to the humeral head and inferior to the distal clavicle
  - Palpate the posterior aspect of the **acromion** and indent skin 2 fingerbreadths medial, 2 fingerbreadths inferior to the posterior acromion
  - This is where you will insert the needle, aiming towards the coracoid process

- ○ Note: this approach will land you in the joint space, but you will probably pierce the labrum in doing so (the US-guided approach avoids this)
- ○ **Procedure**
  - ■ Palpation-guided, clean technique
  - ■ 25 gauge, 1.5-2.5 inch needle
  - ■ Injectate: 4 ml of local anesthetic and 1 ml of corticosteroid (5 ml total)
  - ■ Can also inject prolotherapy, PRP, hyaluronic acid

Palpation-Guided Injections

- ● **Knee Joint Injection**
  - ○ Indicated most commonly for knee osteoarthritis refractory to PT and analgesics
  - ○ Have the patient sitting, knee flexed to 90 degrees
  - ○ Palpate the patellar tendon as it travels inferiorly and attaches to the tibial tuberosity
  - ○ Palpate medial and lateral from there the medial and lateral tibial plateau
  - ○ Mark with your indentation a spot just superior to the tibial plateau on either side of the patellar tendon; this is your injection site
  - ○ **Procedure**
    - ■ Palpation-guided, clean technique
    - ■ 18-22 gauge 1.5-2.5 inch needle
    - ■ Injectate: 3 ml of local anesthetic and 1 ml of corticosteroid
    - ■ Can also inject PRP, hyaluronic acid

Ultrasound-Guided Procedures

- ● Most MSK injections should be done under some form of guidance
- ● Often ultrasound (US) is the most useful form of guidance, due to the ability to detect blood vessels, nerves, or "innocent bystander" structures **and properly avoid them, as well as accurately hit your target**
  - ○ With palpation-guided injections, if the injection doesn't improve the patient's symptoms, you will always wonder, "is it because it just didn't work, or **is it because I didn't actually hit my target?**"
  - ○ There's really no excuse for "nicking a nerve" or causing a large hematoma because you were doing a palpation-guided injection when US would have been the superior method
- ● We will discuss just a few common US-guided procedures, as there is a vast number of procedures with a host of nuances to each, beyond the scope of most PM&R physicians except those interested in USG procedures

Ultrasound Principles

- Ultrasound uses electricity to generate soundwaves (via the piezoelectric effect) which shoot out and bounce back onto the transducer, which converts the soundwaves back into electricity, which gets interpreted by a computer to generate an image based on the pattern of bouncing back by the sound waves

- They do this all as a beam of sound waves that is only as thick as a credit card

- Short axis vs long axis

- In-plane vs. out-of-plane approaches

- Hyperechoic vs. hypoechoic vs. anechoic

Ultrasound Principles

- Arteries vs. veins (both are hollow, dark tubes - use color doppler to help)

- Nerves look like **honeycombs**

- Muscle looks like a slab of steak (speckled appearance / starry sky appearance)

- Tendons have a **linear, fibrillar appearance of striated lines**
    - Tendonitis vs. tendonosis
        - **Tendonitis** = acute inflammatory condition of tendon
        - **Tendonosis** = chronic, degenerative condition of tendon (beyond 3-4 weeks)
            - Tendon is thickened, hypoechoic, with doppler showing neovessels
            - Amenable to regenerative interventions such as PRP, prolotherapy, tendon scraping, high volume injection, percutaneous needle tenotomy

- Bone is bright white

- Fluid (blood, bursa, cyst, inflammation) is dark

Ultrasound-Guided Procedures

- **Shoulder (GHJ) Injection**
    - Patient is side-lying with affected arm adducted (almost like side-sleeping position)
    - Using a 5-12 MHz linear array transducer, scan the posterior shoulder, much like you would palpate the posterior shoulder for a posterior approach palpation-guided shoulder injection
    - Start on the infraspinatus muscle/tendon and follow it onto the greater tuberosity of the humerus
    - This is a great view to visualize the humeral head within the glenoid, with the labrum coming off the glenoid as a fluffy white lip of tissue off the glenoid

- ○ Using US allows you to avoid piercing the labrum
- ○ **Procedure**
  - ■ USG, sterile technique
  - ■ 22 gauge, 2.5 inch needle
  - ■ In-plane, anterior to posterior approach
  - ■ Use 1-5 cc of local anesthetic with a 25 gauge needle, then use local anesthetic in your 22 gauge injection needle, injecting anesthetic as you approach the injection target
  - ■ Once target confirmed with local anesthetic, proceed with injectate
  - ■ Injectate: regenerative, or 4 cc of local anesthetic and 1 cc of corticosteroid (5 cc total)

Ultrasound-Guided Procedures

- ● **Subacromial Subdeltoid Bursa Injection**
  - ○ Patient is seated, arm resting at side
  - ○ Using a 5-12 MHz linear array transducer, scan the area of skin over the deltoid, with part of the probe on the acromion, and the rest of it hanging down in line with the deltoid, in contact with the skin
  - ○ The image will show the deltoid, acromion, supraspinatus tendon, humerus, and subacromial subdeltoid bursa, just superficial to the supraspinatus tendon and just deep to the deltoid and acromion (hence the name)
  - ○ **Procedure**
    - ■ USG, sterile technique
    - ■ 22 gauge, 1.5-2.5 inch needle
    - ■ In-plane approach using the view above
    - ■ Use local anesthetic as discussed before, then guide needle in-plane into the hypoechoic space of the bursa, confirm placement with anesthetic injection, then inject your injectate
    - ■ Injectate: 1 cc of local anesthetic and 1 cc of corticosteroid (2 cc total injectate)

Ultrasound-Guided Procedures

- ● **Neurotoxin injections (botulinum toxin)**
  - ○ Useful for focal spasticity refractory to oral antispasticity medications and splinting, ROM
  - ○ Side effect of dysphagia, weakness
  - ○ Different brands with different doses
  - ○ Use combination of US and EMG guidance for most accurate results
  - ○ Patient positioning depends on the muscle to be injected
    - ■ Always give yourself adequate space for movement of probe and needle
  - ○ **Procedure**

- USG, EMG-guided, clean technique with sterile US gel
- 25-30 gauge, 1.5-2.5 inch injectable EMG needle
- In most cases, identify target muscle, then utilize an out-of-plane technique to confirm placement
- If no motor units are heard on EMG, do not inject that muscle
- Injectate: variable doses of neurotoxin (more units in larger and more spastic muscles)

Fluoroscopic (Xray-Guided) Procedures

- Fluoroscopy is advantageous for most axial spinal injections due to the prohibitive depth of these structures
  - Not optimal for ultrasound; too deep
- Wear radiation protection (lead apron, thyroid shield, glasses)
- These injections generally require multiple views in the AP/lateral/oblique planes in order to accurately approach your target without damaging other structures unnecessarily
- Patients are generally prone or supine with the C-arm above them
- If allergic (not anaphylaxis) to anesthetics, pre-treat with antihistamine +/- oral steroid
- Monitor for side effects or toxicity from the injection
  - Reverse trendelenburg and IV fluids +/- epinephrine are your friend

Fluoroscopic (Xray-Guided) Procedures

- **Epidural Steroid Injection**
  - Indicated for radiculopathy/radiculitis refractory to PT and oral medications, typically in the setting of a herniated disc compressing a spinal nerve root
  - Utilize AP/lateral/oblique views to visualize the needle in 3D space as you approach the target
  - Interlaminar vs. Transforaminal approaches
    - Interlaminar is more of a "shotgun" approach, whereas transforaminal is more precise to a given nerve root
    - **Interlaminar:** pierce the skin between two spinous processes (or two laminae of adjacent levels) and "drop" the needle down, meeting resistance all the way until you pierce the ligamentum flavum and experience **loss of resistance** in the needle (the syringe plunger will depress easily)
      - Loss of resistance confirms placement in the epidural space (just outside the dura)
        - **Epidural** = outside the dura

- o **Intrathecal** = pierce the dura, pierce the subarachnoid space, and you are there, where the CSF circulates (useful for intrathecal baclofen pumps)

Fluoroscopic (Xray-Guided) Procedures

- **Epidural Steroid Injection**
  - o Interlaminar vs. Transforaminal Approaches
    - **Transforaminal:** approach the inferior border of the pedicle with the vertebral body lateral to it, and the inflamed spinal nerve root inferior to your needle as it approaches the inferior border of the pedicle
    - Remember the scottie dog! (on oblique films)
      - Nose = transverse process
      - **Eye = pedicle**
      - Ear = SAP
      - Front leg = IAP
      - Body = lamina
      - Neck = pars interarticularis
  - o Interlaminar approach using contrast will show an epidurogram
  - o Transforaminal approach using contrast will show radiculogram
  - o Inject steroid once confirmed; **dexamethasone is** nonparticulate

Fluoroscopic (Xray-Guided) Procedures

- **Facet Joint Injections**
  - o Useful for diagnostic and therapeutic purposes in facet arthropathy with arthritic facet joint as principal pain generator, refractory to PT and oral medications
  - o The facet joint is a hamburger, a true joint with a joint capsule, articular cartilage, and joint fluid
  - o The joint space is lined up using the C-arm, and the needle is guided into the joint via fluoroscopy
  - o Confirmatory injection of contrast is key prior to injecting medication

- **Medial Branch Block (MBB)**
  - o The medial branches of the dorsal primary rami innervate the facet joints
    - C4-C5 facet (C4 and C5 medial branches); L4-L5 facet (L3 and L4 medial branches)
  - o 2 medial branch blocks are required with at least 80% relief from each one prior to proceeding with a radiofrequency ablation (RFA) of the medial branches
  - o **MBB:** using oblique view, guide needle to junction of SAP and TP, and inject anesthetic

- o **RFA:** guide needle to medial branch, place needle parallel to the nerve, and apply current to it so that it heats up and burns off the medial branch, thus providing longer-lasting (many months) pain relief of that facet joint

Fluoroscopic (Xray-Guided) Procedures

- **SI Joint Injection**
  - o Indicated for SIJ-mediated pain refractory to PT, oral medications, usually in the setting of significant SIJ arthritis
  - o Joint at the junction of the sacrum and ileum
  - o Normally should not have much motion here; hypermobile SIJ is a source of pain, as is an arthritic SIJ
  - o SIJ injection is both diagnostic and therapeutic for SIJ-mediated pain, as even our best physical exam tools for diagnosing the SIJ as a pain generator are just not reliable
  - o The SIJ is typically injected with local anesthetic and steroid to provide long-lasting relief
  - o Patient lies prone as the xray guidance is used to approach the posterior joint line
  - o Use of contrast confirms placement within the joint prior to injecting medication mixture

Fluoroscopic (Xray-Guided) Procedures

- **Spinal Cord Stimulator**
  - o Indicated for **severe**, refractory pain; arachnoiditis, neuropathic pain, CRPS, failed back surgery syndrome (FBSS)
  - o An electrode is implanted near the dorsal horn/posterior column of the level of interest, within the epidural space
  - o Electrical impulses are generated, which stimulate the posterior columns and reduce pain via the **Gate Control Theory**

Fluoroscopic (Xray-Guided) Procedures

- **Stellate Ganglion Block**
  - o This block targets the cervical and thoracic sympathetic ganglia which make up the stellate ganglion
  - o The stellate ganglion is targeted at the **anterior tubercle of the transverse process of C6**
    - ■ This is also called the carotid tubercle due to risk of carotid artery injury
  - o This can actually be done under xray or ultrasound guidance
  - o **This is the gold standard test for confirming CRPS**
  - o It is also therapeutic for CRPS in combination with noninvasive treatments
  - o A positive block relieves the patient's CRPS pain and causes an ipsilateral Horner syndrome

Intrathecal Baclofen Pump Refills

- Refer to SCI (spasticity section) for detailed discussion on baclofen pumps
- Intrathecal baclofen (ITB) pumps are generally refilled by the PM&R physician every 1-6 months
- ITB pumps all have different alarms that will sound loudly in case of **low medication** or **empty pump** status
  - IN GENERAL
    - **Low medication amount:** the pump will beep a single beep at regular intervals
      - Patient is educated at this point to call their doctor or attend their scheduled meeting (these are usually scheduled in anticipation of pump alarm dates)
    - **Empty pump:** either the pump ran out of medication or the catheter is kinked, etc.; the pump will sound a two-tone alarm at regular intervals, which is a **pump emergency**
      - Patient is educated to go to the ED at this point, or be seen emergently in clinic for refill
      - Oral baclofen often substitutes here to buy time until the pump can be refilled

Intrathecal Baclofen Pump Refills

- **Refilling ITB pump procedure**
  - The pump is "interrogated" using an electronic interrogation device that wirelessly communicates with the ITB pump in the vicinity of the patient
  - The interrogation data will inform the physician how much baclofen is expected to be in the pump at this point (once you withdraw all the medication before injecting the new batch)
  - It will also tell you the total daily dose and the dosing schedule (simple continuous vs. boluses throughout the day/night), reservoir volume, expected alarm dates, drug concentration
  - Once interrogated, the drainage and refill procedure is begun, using a sterile refill kit with sterile gloves
  - Once skin over the pump is sterilized, a sterile drape is placed over the procedure site
  - The pump orientation is palpated, and a pump guide is used to tell you where the central port access point is
  - A needle is used to pierce the access port and empty the contents of the pump into your syringe
    - The volume you withdraw should equal the expected volume from your interrogation!

- o Keep needle in place and switch out the syringe for your "new batch" medication syringe
- o Inject new batch of baclofen, then reprogram the pump settings using the interrogation device
- o Print out new parameters, including alarm dates, for you and patient, then document parameters in your note

*Remember: procedures are hard, and **nobody** is immediately good at them. It takes a long time of being bad at procedures before you are kind of, somewhat, confident with them. Remember this when you watch someone else perform a procedure effortlessly. It took them a LOT of practice to be able to do that.*

Chapter 25: Getting Ready to Practice

Disclaimer: This chapter is not intended as actual, individual, specific career or financial advice, and should not be taken that way. Dr. D'Angelo is not a financial or career advice professional, and the content in this chapter (and in this entire book) is intended purely for educational purposes, and not actual, actionable advice.

Starting the Job Search

- In the late summer/early fall of your PGY4 or fellowship year (or 2nd fellowship year for peds fellows), you will start your job search for your first attending job

- **Congratulations!** It took a lot to get this far

- So, where do you start?

- Think about what **type of practice** and **location** options you want to pursue
    - Private practice? Academic? Solo? Multispecialty group? Hospital-based? Clinic-based?
    - Inpatient? Outpatient? Part-time? Full-time?
    - Employee? Independent Contractor?
    - Procedures? No procedures?
    - Like working with residents and medical students? Enjoy teaching?
    - Rural? Urban? Densely populated city?
    - Low cost of living? High cost of living?

- Some people say, "location, lifestyle, money: pick two"
    - Really, it's more grey than that

Practice Options

- **Private practice**
    - In general, more $$$ potential, but potentially more work
        - Need to generate more volume, work more hours
        - Or, choose to scale back and make less money
    - "Be your own boss"
        - Choose the staff in your practice
        - Set your own hours
    - Riskier option
        - 100% "eat what you kill"
        - Utterly dependent on referrals, marketing, word of mouth, reputation
        - May or may not come with a benefits package
    - If group practice, after 2-3 years, option for buy-in
        - Typically a 6-figure amount that allows you to purchase ownership of the practice
        - Potential for much higher income with partnership

- ○ This is the true entrepreneurial, "business of medicine" option

Practice Options

- ● **Academic Practice**
  - ○ More predictable, structured form of practice
  - ○ Typically salaried with incentive structure in place (RVUs and other levers that you can pull to generate yourself more income)
  - ○ Teaching residents and medical students is a routine part of practice
  - ○ Not your own boss
    - ■ Little to no control over hours and staff hiring/firing
    - ■ There is always someone higher up you will answer to
  - ○ Stable, guaranteed income
    - ■ In general, less $$$ than private practice
  - ○ Can have a robust benefits package, which itself can bring huge financial value

Practice Options

- ● **Part-time vs. full-time**
  - ○ Full-time = more money, more hours, more benefits
  - ○ Part-time = less money, fewer hours, potentially no benefits
    - ■ Typical for employers to require 60-75% time to qualify for benefits package

- ● **Location: low cost of living vs. high cost of living**
  - ○ Low COL = "less attractive area", "fewer things to do", can be FAR cheaper, meaning more $$$ in your pocket
  - ○ High COL = "more attractive area", "more things to do", can be FAR more expensive, meaning less $$$ in your pocket
  - ○ Want to live near family? Away from family?
  - ○ Consider if you want to live in a state with no state income tax

Searching for a Job

- ● Once you've figured out what type of job you are looking for, now it's time to begin the search

- ● Make sure your CV is updated with relevant information
  - ○ Professional photo on CV is a nice touch
  - ○ +/- cover letter

- ● How do you do this?

- ● Options include internet searches, signing up on online physician job boards, cold-calling practices, cold-emailing practices, asking your attendings for contacts, and attending national conferences where there are job fairs and other networking options

- ○ Always bring your interview suit to conferences for this reason!
- Wait for the flurry of offers to interview you

Applying and Interviewing for Jobs

- If you like a job description on paper, once the employer or recruiter emails or calls you, it's time to schedule a phone interview (or in-person interview, if at a conference)
- Prepare an introductory or "mission statement" that represents you and what you want to accomplish in your practice
  - ○ The type of practice setting you're looking for, the type of patients and pathologies you want to treat, inpatient vs. outpatient, procedures or no procedures, etc.
- This is essentially a "feeler" interview in which both parties gauge whether or not this is a good general fit
  - ○ "Heavy" questions should not be asked at this time
    - ■ E.g. "Could we get rid of the non-compete clause?"
    - ■ E.g. "How much can I expect to make?"
      - Usually you know a general range, as it's commonly included in the job posting, but this is not the time to be asking hard, uncomfortable specifics like that

Interviewing for Jobs

- If you and the employer both like what you hear during the initial "feeler" interview, then a second interview will be scheduled
- The second interview may be another phone interview, but often the employer will invite you to fly/drive out and spend 1-2 days interviewing and taking in the practice
  - ○ The employer typically pays for your travel and lodging
- If you are not "wowed" by the job on the initial interview, it still may not be a bad idea to attend the second interview, as you may discover that you actually like the job, and details about this job can be used as leverage with other jobs during negotiations

Interviewing for Jobs

- The second interview is more of a "getting to know you" interview
- Questions about how you might handle certain situations may arise
- Deeper questions may also arise, such as how many patients per day you will be expected to see, further details on the structure of your day, further details on your daily duties, benefits details, etc.
- After the second interview, if both of you are at least somewhat interested in each other, they may send you an offer

The Contract

- Congratulations! Interviews went well, and you have been mailed or emailed a contract offer
- It will include pages and pages of legalese, including all the details of your contract
    - Salary, benefits, duties, expectations, vacation, etc.
- Hire a medical contract lawyer
    - Ask if they have a resident or fellow discount
    - They will usually charge hourly, and it can be well worth the price
    - They will thoroughly peruse the contract and give you points of discussion you can use for negotiations
    - Often, academic practices will not change anything about their contracts

The Contract

- Now it's time to think about negotiations
- These may take place over the phone, over email, or in person
    - You are not obligated to conduct these in strictly one setting
        - If you prefer email to gather your thoughts appropriately, then do that
        - If you prefer phone / in person in order to convey your thoughts more accurately, then do that

Negotiations

- Anything goes!
- Nothing is off the table
    - If you really want it, ask for it
- You are worth A LOT
- If you want something, ask for it, or you will regret it, despise yourself, and build resentment towards your employer
    - If they say no, *no sweat!* They said no. Feel relieved and proud that you at least asked
- You are selling your education, skillset, financial value to them, and your personality
    - These are all valuable assets

How to Negotiate

- **It's all about how you say it**
    - "I want to work less so I can play at home."
    - VS.
    - "80% time would allow me to strike the right work-life balance that will keep me satisfied and energized at work."

- **Bring data with you to back up your counteroffers**
  - Print out the latest income reports from different organizations, representing the ranges, median, max, etc. incomes for your particular practice type around the country
  - Inform your counteroffers with these data, to show that you're not just "making the numbers up"
- **If you don't want to answer a question (e.g. what's your $number?), then say you prefer not to disclose that at this time**
  - Make them make the first offer
  - You don't ever have to tell them "your number"

How to Negotiate

- **What to negotiate for**
  - More money (either guaranteed or via incentives), signing bonus, relocation bonus
  - More/better benefits
  - More vacation time
  - Parking space, office location
  - Hiring and firing power
  - Call vs. no call
  - Removing the non-compete clause, or reducing its radius or duration
  - How much notice they require from you before you quit
  - How much notice they have to give you if they want to terminate you
  - Research requirement vs. no requirement
- **All of this is fair game**
- All of this requires tact in how you say it
- Always be friendly and thankful; "kill them with kindness"

How to Negotiate

- **Negotiations are uncomfortable, and that's normal**
  - If it's not uncomfortable, you might not be asking for enough
- **Nothing actually bad will happen if you ask them for something**
  - Either they say no, in which case, at least you feel satisfied that you asked
  - Or they say no, and now we are offended that you asked that, and now we don't want you
    - In this case, **GOOD!** You just dodged a bullet! Good thing you figured this out now, rather than 1 year down the line.
- **Think** like a cold mercenary, but **act** like the charming, bright, cheerful person you are

- "But I'm shy and reserved"
  - So am I
  - PRACTICE, and it will become second nature
  - Remember, you are HIGHLY VALUABLE

Financial Health and Literacy

- Congratulations! You've signed your contract. Now what do you do with your money?
- Well, what are your financial goals in life? Where do you want to be when you retire?
- Most physicians will have similar goals
  - Build wealth (i.e. "become as rich as possible")
  - Financial security (i.e. "never have to worry about money")
  - Ensure financial security for your family or children if you plan to have them
  - Maybe buy some toys along the way, donate to charity, and take nice vacations
  - Do all of this while paying the least amount of taxes
- Sound complicated? It's not. And **you can do it yourself.**
  - The financial industry wants you to think it's complicated so that you have to pay them to handle your finances

Saving Money (Purchasing Wealth)

- When you get your first paycheck, typically an electronic direct deposit into your bank account, it's going to be a huge amount of money compared to what you have seen in the past
- You will feel lulled into a false sense of "being rich", and will have the huge temptation to spend it without regard, "since there's so much of it!"
  - This comes in the form of a new, big house, fancy car, huge brand new TV, etc.
- You need to **AVOID this lifestyle inflation if you want to build wealth**
  - Also called lifestyle creep, as it often happens very gradually
  - "Live like a resident" for at least a few years
    - **This DOES NOT mean suffering!**

Saving Money (Purchasing Wealth)

- Ok, so you're convinced that saving money is a good idea
- Where do I save my money? How do I save it? How much do I save?
- You can withdraw it from your checking account and have the cash on hand, then stuff it under your mattress or keep it in a closet
  - Your money is with you at all times
  - But it can be stolen, destroyed in a house fire, etc.
  - **It also won't grow if it's just sitting there**

- The US dollar undergoes inflation at a rate of roughly 2% each year
- That means your money needs to grow at a rate of 2% each year **just for you to simply keep pace with inflation** and maintain the same actual value of your money
- Thus, it's bad if your money doesn't grow at all (keeping it all in cash in your closet), and it's bad if your money only grows to keep pace with inflation (hard to build wealth at a 2% growth rate)

- So how do we actually grow our money to outpace inflation?
  - You invest in the stock market with a **reasonable investing plan**

Saving Money (Purchasing Wealth)

- Before you invest your money, you need to follow some sort of reasonable algorithm for what to do with your money

- Do you have bills to pay? Set aside money for this before investing

- Do you have an emergency fund set up containing 3-6 months of living expenses?
  - Flat tires, car repairs, weather damage to home, hospital expenses, lost job, etc.

- Set aside money for this in an easy-to-access account before investing
  - A reasonable place to save this money is in a high-yield savings account, which typically has interest rates in the 2-2.5% range
  - You can also do certificates of deposit (CDs)

- Do you have student loans? Mortgage? Set aside money to pay these
  - In general, pay off the highest interest item first, then the next highest

- Ok, now let's invest and **build wealth**

Investing

- Investing sounds intimidating, but the fundamentals are simple, and **if you can get through medical school and residency, you can invest your money**

- You want to set aside **at least 20%** of every paycheck to go straight into your retirement contributions (i.e., invest it)
  - 50% is achievable for many physicians, due to our high incomes, and will lead to more wealth and an earlier retirement, if those are your goals

- There are different retirement accounts you can invest in; let's talk about them
  - Individual retirement account (IRA), 401(k), 403(b), 457(b), taxable account

Individual Retirement Account (IRA)

- This is an account you can set up at your bank or other online investing firm

- It's an account designed to get people to save for retirement by offering them tax advantages for putting money into it

- Each individual is allowed their own IRA (couples can't co-own a single IRA - each person must have their own under their own name alone)
- You can contribute up to $6,000 annually into your IRA (in 2019)
  - Great...what's the big deal? I can do that in a savings account, too
- A traditional IRA lets you **deduct that $6,000 from your income tax**
- A Roth IRA has you pay income tax on it now, but **withdraw it tax-free when you retire**
- You choose what type of stock market funds to invest the money in
  - We will discuss how to select funds later in this section

401(k), 403(b), 457(b)

- These are employer retirement accounts/plans offered to employees
- The annual limit for how much you can contribute is $19,000 per year per person for total 401(k) and 403(b) contributions, and separate $19,000 per year per person into the 457(b) pool
  - These also come in **Traditional and Roth varieties**
- Employers offer these because it makes them attractive to potential employees
- Employers typically **match your contributions dollar-for-dollar** with contributions of their own, **giving you free money** (up to a certain % of contributions)
  - This is why most people say contribute here to get the maximum match before deciding on contributing to your IRA
- You have to choose what funds you want this money to be invested into once you've contributed the money
  - Your employer will offer you a selection of funds to choose from

Taxable Investing (Brokerage) Account

- This is just what it sounds like; unlike IRAs and 401ks (in which you don't get taxed on the growth of your money), in taxable brokerage accounts, you get taxed as your money grows
  - **Capital Gains Tax**
    - If your brokerage account does really well in a certain year, you will pay taxes on some percentage of those gains
- Basically, it is an effective way to build wealth, **and it should be utilized,** but only after exhausting the $6,000 and $19,000 limits of your tax-advantaged retirement accounts
- Thus, if you are in a position where you are cursing the fact that you are paying capital gains taxes, **you are in a good position and should feel good**

529 Plan

- This is pretty much what people refer to when they refer to a "trust fund" for their children, although truthfully a trust fund is a different thing

- A 529 plan is a state-sponsored savings account that people typically use for saving for their children's college expenses

- Why not just use a savings account or simply save this money in a taxable investing account?
  - Because it won't grow enough in the savings account (remember, it gets to grow over a period of about 18 years!)
  - And because if you use 529 funds to pay for your children's college expenses, you don't have to pay taxes on it!
    - You still pay your own federal income tax on this money, but when you withdraw it from the 529 plan and use it to pay for your children's college tuition, etc., you do not have to pay taxes on that withdrawal

529 Plan

- Do I have to use my own state's 529 plan?
  - No! You can live in Oregon, send your kids to school in Idaho, and use Vermont's 529 plan
  - You should consider your own state's 529 plan because it may offer you income tax deductions as reward for using their plan

- Otherwise, it's just like any other investment account
  - You pick one account per child (typically), designate them as the single beneficiary of the account, and invest it in reasonable investment options depending on how old they are

- Some states have "better" plans than others, depending on costs and investment options

- You can contribute up to $15,000 per year per child ($30,000 per child for couples filing jointly), but beyond that, you have to report it to the government when you do your taxes, as there is a federal gift tax you have to pay if you gift your child >$15,000 in a single year

What Do I Actually Invest In?

- Isn't the stock market risky/stupid?
  - It is risky, but you generally want this risk at this early stage of your career

- Stocks are ownership shares of a given company
  - If you purchase stock of a company, you own a little bit of that company

- A reliable, reasonable way to invest your money and watch it grow steadily (slowly but surely) over time is to invest in index funds

- **Index funds** allow you to invest in the stock of hundreds of companies at once by buying a very small share of each company

- ○ You can purchase an index fund of **the entire stock market**
- ○ You can purchase an index fund of just tech companies
- ○ You can purchase an index fund of just clothing companies
- This is reasonable so that you avoid putting all your eggs in one basket, e.g. only investing in one "hot company"

What Do I Actually Invest In?

- **Bond Index Fund**
  - ○ A bond is basically a legal agreement that you are lending money to a company, or city, or government, with the idea that they will pay you interest on that loan until the term of the loan is over
    - ■ E.g. a city may want to build some new roads, and issue a bond out that people like you can purchase to finance it; they will pay you interest on your loan
  - ○ Bonds are more predictable, less volatile, and less risky
    - ■ As such, they pay somewhere in the 2-4% interest range
    - ■ Thus, **less risk, but also less reward**
      - Whereas **the stock market is high risk, high reward**
  - ○ A bond index fund is an index fund of a lot of different bonds
    - ■ Why not pick one bond instead of a whole index? Same reason as for stock index funds: you want to NOT put all your eggs in one basket; you want to diversify your investments so that you can weather any storm or economic downturn

How Much Do I Invest in Stocks vs. Bonds?

- This is called **asset allocation**; i.e. deciding what percentage of your money you should invest in stocks, and what percentage in bonds
  - ○ Your money is your assets; how are you going to allocate your money (your assets)?
- A general rule of thumb is to take (100 - your age), and this is the amount you should allocate towards stocks (if you are 30, you should allocate 70% of your investments into stock index funds)
  - ○ This leaves 30% for bond index fund(s)
- As you age closer to retirement, your investments should gradually shift to less risky investments, such as bonds
  - ○ This way, if the market takes a huge hit (like the 2008 recession), you will be relatively unaffected, and can retire with all your money intact as planned
  - ○ If the market takes a huge hit, and you're 32 with all your money in stocks, YOU WILL RECOVER, because you have the next 20-40 years of stock market growth to ride

Ride the Waves

- Over your career, by following a reasonable asset allocation based on your age until retirement, you will see your money ride high and grow immensely with stock market upswings, and dip down tremendously, watching your money disappear

- This is scary, but if you simply **stay the course** and follow your reasonable asset allocation and investment strategy, your money will grow reliably over time

- **Do not panic sell when the market downturns and your money is disappearing**

- If you simply continue investing in your total stock market and total bond market index funds as planned, you will most likely recover well

- Over 20-40 years, the total stock market will dip and rise endlessly
    - Sometimes the dips are huge, and sometimes the rises are huge (bear vs. bull market)
    - However, **over the long run** (20-40 years) it will have grown substantially
    - Thus, if you stay in the entire stock market for 20-40 years, you will see growth

But Can't I Invest in Other Things?

- Sure!

- You can invest in real estate by purchasing properties yourself and being a landlord, collecting rent from your tenants
    - This is not passive, however, and essentially is an entire job by itself
    - However, it can definitely be a path toward financial independence and wealth
    - But it is not passive until the late stages (after years and years of collecting properties and rent)

- You can invest in single companies, gold, silver, bitcoin, the latest hot stock

- But **the vast majority of the time, you will not outperform passive index funds**
    - Period.

Retirement

- As you get closer toward retirement, you should shift your money gradually out of the market, and into more secure (but less payoff) investments, such as bonds

- Thus, your money is a lot safer, and should not change much

- If you have a lot of money in Roth accounts (Roth IRA, Roth 401(k)), you can withdraw this tax-free!

- But in general you want to touch your taxable money first, since you are paying capital gains taxes on it as it grows, while the Roth money, it can just grow and grow and grow, completely tax-free, so you generally want to withdraw the Roth money last (or save it for your children, grandchildren, etc.)

Retirement

- When you reach age 70.5, you are actually required to start withdrawing money from traditional IRAs, Roth and traditional 401(k)s, 403(b)s, and 457(b)s
  - These are called required minimum distributions (RMDs)
  - Roth IRAs actually don't require you to withdraw any money from it until the account owner dies

- **How much do I withdraw?**
  - There is a generally agreed upon **safe withdrawal rate of about 4%** of your entire portfolio
  - This means you can withdraw 4% of your entire net worth to live off each year, and not actually touch any of your principal investment (in other words, **you are living off the interest** of your investments)
  - For example, if you own $1,000,000, theoretically you can safely withdraw $40,000 per year and live off that alone, without causing your wealth to shrink
  - Some people like to play it safe and withdraw somewhere between 3-4% instead of at 4%
  - It all depends on personal risk tolerance

You've Won

- If you've managed to save 20-50% of your income as a physician into a reasonable investing portfolio (i.e. wealth-building portfolio) over your entire career, then you've done a fantastic job and should be proud

- You should be able to accomplish this and still enjoy life
  - Maybe not buy a Ferrari, but still enjoy life while not feeling inhibited

- Having this level of financial security and financial independence (i.e. not having to work to live) will allow you to **choose** how much you want to work, thus preventing burnout, and giving you increased satisfaction as a doctor

- Having this level of financial security will make you a better doctor, a better spouse, a better parent, a better friend, a better softball league teammate, a better board game partner, and a happier, more fulfilled person

If you've just completed this entire book, you're phenomenal! And if you've only read this chapter, well, I think you're phenomenal, too!

Now go be the best physiatrist you can be.

-Alex D'Angelo, M.D.

References, Corrections, and Updates

For complete list of textbook and video series references, corrections, and updates to content, please refer to the corresponding webpage at:

https://www.pmrrecap.com/referencesandcorrections

Made in the USA
Middletown, DE
13 January 2022

58543544R00150